PREGNANCY HACKS

PREGNANCY HACKS

350+ Easy Hacks for a Happy and Healthy Pregnancy!

AMANDA SHAPIN MICHELSON

ADAMS MEDIA
New York London Toronto Sydney New Delhi

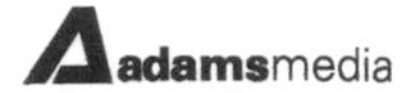

Adams Media
An Imprint of Simon & Schuster, Inc.
100 Technology Center Drive
Stoughton, Massachusetts 02072

First Adams Media trade paperback edition December 2020

ADAMS MEDIA and colophon are trademarks of Simon & Schuster.

For information about special discounts for bulk purchases, please contact Simon & Schuster Special Sales at 1-866-506-1949 or business@simonandschuster.com.

The Simon & Schuster Speakers Bureau can bring authors to your live event. For more information or to book an event contact the Simon & Schuster Speakers Bureau at 1-866-248-3049 or visit our website at www.simonspeakers.com.

Interior design and illustrations by Priscilla Yuen

Manufactured in the United States of America

3 2022

Library of Congress Cataloging-in-Publication Data
Names: Michelson, Amanda Shapin, author.
Title: Pregnancy hacks / Amanda Shapin Michelson.
Description: First Adams Media trade paperback edition. | Avon, Massachusetts: Adams Media, 2020. | Series: Hacks | Includes index.
Identifiers: LCCN 2020034712 | ISBN 9781507214572 (pb) | ISBN 9781507214589 (ebook)
Subjects: LCSH: Pregnancy--Popular works.
Classification: LCC RG525 .M448 2020 | DDC 618.2--dc23
LC record available at https://lccn.loc.gov/2020034712

ISBN 978-1-5072-1457-2
ISBN 978-1-5072-1458-9 (ebook)

This book is intended as general information only, and should not be used to diagnose or treat any health condition. In light of the complex, individual, and specific nature of health problems, this book is not intended to replace professional medical advice. The ideas, procedures, and suggestions in this book are intended to supplement, not replace, the advice of a trained medical professional. Consult your physician before adopting any of the suggestions in this book, as well as about any condition that may require diagnosis or medical attention. The author and publisher disclaim any liability arising directly or indirectly from the use of this book.

To my daughter, Millie,
for making me a mama.

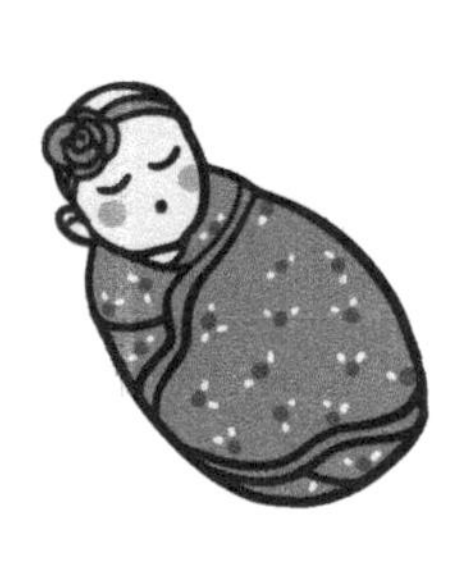

CONTENTS

ACKNOWLEDGMENTS

There are so many people I want to thank for helping to bring this book to life. First, to all the moms that came before me and lent their expertise and personal experiences, thank you. Your guidance will undoubtedly bring comfort and strength to many expectant parents out there.

A huge thank you to my husband, Matt, who has supported me during every step of this process. He was the inspiration behind "Partner Hacks," as he was the perfect partner during my pregnancy and was the perfect partner as I wrote this book.

Special love and thanks to my baby girl, Millie. You made me a mom and gave me the greatest role I could ever hope for. It's because of you that I found the passion to share my stories around pregnancy and motherhood. And thank you for being such a good sleeper, allowing me to write this book during your naps and after bedtime. Also, love and thanks to our pup, Ollie, for your companionship and cuddles while I wrote.

Thank you to my parents, Alice and Paul, who have always believed in me and been eager to read and edit my work. I'm pretty sure my mom has expected me to write a book since I was in elementary school, and I'm grateful this dream is becoming a reality (for both of us).

Thank you to the rest of the Shapin and Michelson families for all of the support you've given me.

And a heartfelt thank you to the women who helped me navigate my own pregnancy and shared their insights for this book. These women are doctors, therapists, psychologists, yoga instructors, social workers, teachers—many more things—and moms. They shared their professional and personal advice, helping to form more than 350 hacks that I now get to share with you. Some are mothers, some not, but all of these women shared their wisdom, support, love, and excitement during the writing process. Thank you to Lauren Acker, Sydney Berkowitz, Amy Cowen, Sarah Ezrin, Shira (& Noah) Hichenberg, Robyn Isman, Julia Kraft, Caryn LoCastro, Jill Lubochinski, Sara Onufer, Carroll Ratpojanakul, Lianna Semegran, Jackie Shapin, Alison Silverman, Yaffa Tilles, Michele Weisz, and Anna

Wolfson. Thank you to Jodi Farrera, my midwife and leader of the group I attended during my own pregnancy, for making the experience a pretty fun one.

Thank you to the team at *The Everymom* for giving me an outlet to share my stories on motherhood and for creating a much-needed space to support and celebrate all mothers.

Thank you to Julia Jacques, Laura Daly, and the rest of Adams Media for the opportunity to write this book and for all the support along the way. And thank you to my agent, Leigh Eisenman, for her expert guidance.

Women are truly so strong, bringing life into the world, and this book celebrates women while keeping them comfortable and happy through pregnancy. To all the moms and soon-to-be-moms, thank you for reading this book and bringing me along on your journey to motherhood.

INTRODUCTION

You're pregnant! Congratulations and welcome to this very exciting time in your life. These next nine months (actually, it's officially ten months from start to finish) are going to be a wild ride.

Everyone experiences pregnancy in a different way, and parts of it may not be the most comfortable or easy time for you. While pregnancy is a beautiful experience, it may also come with physical discomfort, sleepless nights (yes, even before the baby arrives), feelings of anxiety, concerns about what to eat (or not eat), and a whole host of other concerns. After all, growing a human in your belly is no easy feat! But don't worry; that's where *Pregnancy Hacks* comes in: to make all three trimesters a bit easier and more pleasant, with hundreds of simple tips. This book will provide creative solutions for the challenging and uncomfortable parts of pregnancy. Here are some examples:

- Pants feeling too tight? Flip to Chapter 2 to find ways to extend the life of your current clothes before buying maternity options.
- Heartburn bothering you nonstop? Chapter 3 gives you surefire ways to avoid it.
- Struggling to focus at work? Check out tips for battling pregnancy brain in Chapter 4.
- Feeling overwhelmed as you create your registry? Head to Chapter 5 for secrets to asking for everything you need—and nothing you don't.
- Unsure of how to prepare for your first days at home with your baby? Chapter 6 has everything you need to feel ready, physically and mentally.

Whatever answers you're looking for, this book has the tools and support you deserve. You'll even find a special section in each chapter that provides tips for your partner, allowing them to be extra helpful to you on your pregnancy journey. Pass this book along to them, and they will be prepared to successfully support you, without you having to ask. Remember, you are in this together!

Everyone has a totally unique pregnancy, so you can use this book however it works best for you. Seek out the chapters and hacks that you need, when you need them, or read the book all the way through, highlighting or marking tips that you want to use.

Your pregnancy is just the beginning of the most amazing adventure: parenthood. Let these hacks put your mind and body at ease so you can focus on your baby and yourself.

CHAPTER 1

Navigating the Early Weeks of Pregnancy

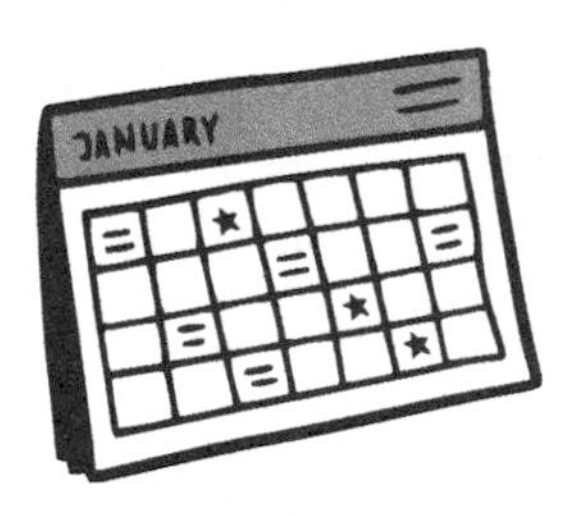

Welcome to the beginning of your pregnancy! This is an exciting time, but it can also be a bit nerve racking. While you have something so huge happening, you may be keeping your pregnancy news quiet, perhaps not ready to share with extended family, friends, and coworkers. Not openly talking about your pregnancy can make the first few weeks of pregnancy and the first trimester feel even more uneasy. Since you may not feel comfortable reaching out to your friends with your pregnancy questions, you might need help with questions that pop into your mind—this chapter is here to help! It's normal to have a lot of questions, especially if this is your first baby. In this chapter, you'll find helpful hacks and tips as you begin your pregnancy journey, including advice for the first things to check off your pregnancy to-do list, ideas on how to hide your pregnancy (if that's what you've decided to do), plus suggestions for staying healthy and positive during the first trimester.

1 Join a local parents' group online to get recommendations. Check out various social media channels to find a local group of parents who can offer advice on nearby healthcare providers, practices, hospitals, birthing centers, pediatricians, and other topics. They may already have information on popular topics archived, or you can post a new question. Everyone will have their own opinion, of course, but the top local options will likely get lots of recommendations.

••◆••

2 Keep an open mind to all the care and delivery options available in your area. Do you see yourself delivering in a hospital, at a birthing center, or at home? Will you see an ob-gyn, a midwife, and/or a doula? Do some research and see what you and your partner will be most comfortable with. You may have always pictured a hospital birth, but that isn't the only option, and learning about the other possibilities may open your eyes to a new preference. See what options are available in your area and discuss these with your partner and your doctor. Aim to decide early so your birth prep can align with your preferences.

3 Interview multiple doctors before choosing a practice. You are going to see your doctor or midwife a lot over the next nine months. Make sure your personalities are in sync, that they aren't rushing through your appointments, and you feel comfortable with them. Also, check the likelihood that they will be the one to deliver your baby. Many practices are large, and you often end up with the doctor "on call," not your personal OB, when you go into labor. You'll likely have a lot of questions and concerns over the course of your pregnancy and you will want a provider and/or a group practice that you trust and can confide in. Ask several doctors a few questions about their philosophy until you find one who is a good fit for you.

• • ♦ • •

4 Tell your doctor and any ultrasound technicians at each appointment if you don't want to know the sex of the baby. If you do decide to keep the sex a surprise, remind your provider and any ultrasound technicians that you meet with at the beginning of your appointments. Though most are very careful, you don't want them accidentally spilling the news during your visit!

5 Schedule your first round of appointments all at once and close to the same time. Once you take an at-home pregnancy test and get the positive result, call your doctor to schedule your first appointment. Usually that first visit will be when you are around eight weeks pregnant. Some offices have busy schedules and hard-to-get appointment slots, so call for yours as soon as you get that positive test. And when you're at that first appointment, see if you can schedule the next few months' worth of appointments at once to avoid having to schedule another one each time. It might also be a good idea to make them at the same time—for example, the second Wednesday of the month—so you and others know when to expect them. Even if you end up needing to reschedule a few, it's easier to have them set in advance. Write down or enter all your appointments in your calendar so you don't forget and so you can properly plan ahead.

6 When you're ready to share, talk about your company's policies with a coworker who has already taken maternity leave. When you are comfortable discussing your pregnancy with someone at work, ask a fellow coworker who has been through it if they have any tips about navigating maternity leave. They may have some ideas or suggestions that will work for your situation as well.

• • ♦ • •

7 Don't assume you need to take every prenatal test. Your doctor will probably mention various tests that are available to you—but you don't have to take them all! Some are standard, some are elective, some are invasive, and some may come with a big price tag if they're not fully covered by insurance. Request a full list of available tests from your doctor and see which ones they recommend for you. Review and discuss with your partner to decide what is best for your situation and schedule these accordingly.

8 Make a pro/con list about finding out the sex of the baby. Chat with your partner and decide if you want to be surprised by the baby's sex at the birth, or if you'd prefer to find out in advance. Some say that waiting until the birth is one of the last big surprises you can experience in life. Others prefer to know in advance, as it allows them to decorate the nursery and buy certain clothes and products and choose only one baby name. Some parents-to-be even say that finding out the gender in advance makes them feel closer to the developing baby. It's a personal decision, so do what feels best to you.

• • ♦ • •

9 Call your insurance company to ask all your pregnancy- and baby-related coverage questions. As you celebrate the big news of pregnancy, there are fewer fun logistics to work through, like insurance. Review your plan and understand what is covered, including appointments, genetic and/or prenatal testing, and details related to labor and delivery.

10 Stay on top of your finances by scheduling a meeting with a financial advisor. Sit down with your partner and a financial advisor to talk through the costs of a baby and how that will impact your finances now and in the future. Create a savings plan that works for your family and put it into practice before the baby arrives.

• • ♦ • •

11 During your first trimester, get a handle on your postpartum benefits. Gather documents online and from your employer to review short-term disability, maternity leave, and FMLA (Family and Medical Leave Act) options. Laws vary by state and by company size; see what is offered where you live and where you work. Know your rights and figure out what the best course of action will be for you. This information will impact your finances and your childcare decisions, so learning what you have now will help you make informed choices.

Creative Ways to Hide Your Pregnancy from Others

You're probably excited about your pregnancy and can't wait to share the big news. But if you're keeping it a secret in the first trimester, here are some ways to keep your secret, even if you have plans to meet your best friends for after-work drinks.

12 **Design your own mocktails.** Brainstorm what your favorite go-to cocktail might look like as a tasty mocktail so you have an order ready to go.

13 **Arrive first.** When meeting friends at a bar, get there first and order your mocktail before your friends arrive. This will fool your friends into thinking that you are drinking and will make your night more enjoyable thanks to a well-crafted virgin cocktail.

14 **Give the bartender a heads-up.** Slip away from your friends and chat with the friendliest bartender you see. Let them know you want virgin drinks, no matter what you actually order or what your friends might order for you.

15 **Order the same thing as your partner.** When out with a group, order the same drink as your partner. When they are almost done with their drink and no one is looking, switch your glasses. Suddenly it seems like you've been keeping up with the rest of the group even though you haven't had a sip.

16 **Ask the bartender for a taste of wine.** Get to the bar early and ask the bartender to taste a wine on the menu, but then don't take a sip. Hang on to your taster of wine, which to anyone else will look like an almost-finished glass of wine. Once your friends arrive, they will see your nearly empty wineglass and assume you're one glass in.

17 **Sip from a Solo cup.** When hosting friends, use Solo cups or other opaque cup options. Guests won't be able to see whether you have water or wine in your cup.

18 **Claim food poisoning.** It's not the most glamorous illness to come down with, but it's a good match for morning sickness in a pinch. It explains vomiting and provides a continued excuse as to why you're avoiding sushi and alcohol.

19 **Make diet-inspired excuses.** If your friends are skeptical as to why you are skipping soft cheeses and wine, say you are trying out a Paleo lifestyle or are doing a Whole30 challenge. Both diets do not allow dairy or alcohol.

20 **Fake a fitness challenge.** If you're at least semi-athletic, tell your friends you're training for a big race, perhaps a marathon. And if you are not athletic, say you've got your sights set on completing your first 5k. With such an exciting goal, you have a set reason why you can't stay out late and are skipping alcohol: You need to stay well rested and clearheaded for your early-morning training runs!

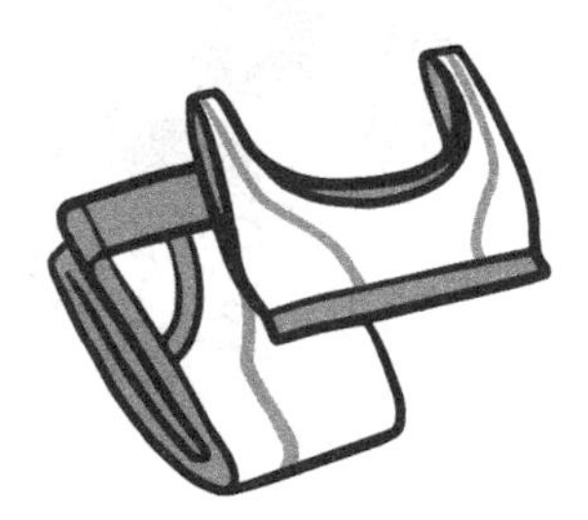

21 **Work your angles for social media to hide your bump.** Want to continue posting to social media but your growing belly is a giveaway to the secret that you're hiding? Play around with your angles and continue snapping until you find a shot that casually conceals your belly. Pictures shot from behind of you looking off into the distance are a good cover-up. Holding props or a bag in front of you can come in handy as well. Or just shoot from the neck up. If that's not working, post throwback photos.

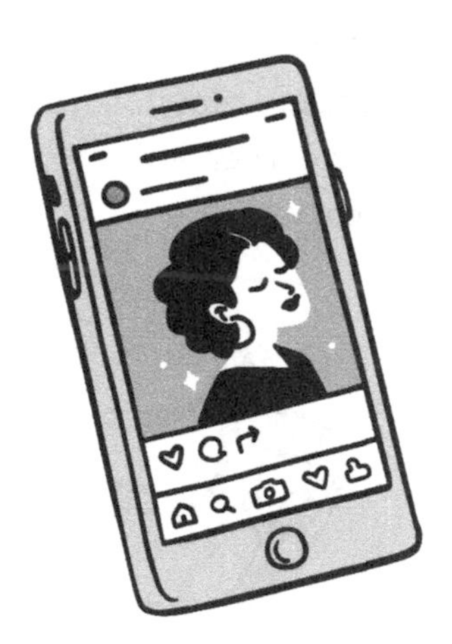

22 Program important medical numbers in your/your partner's phone. It's common for many questions to arise in the early weeks of pregnancy. When concerns arise, don't hesitate to reach out to your doctor. In your phone, save the phone number for your doctor's office and/or the nurse hotline for easy access. Save your doctor's email or a link to their online forum if that's the preferred method of communication. Have your partner do the same.

•••◆•••

23 Upgrade your medicine cabinet to include pregnancy-safe medications. Hopefully you're feeling as good as possible during the first few weeks and months of pregnancy, but know that some of your go-to remedies for everyday annoyances like colds, headaches, allergies, and so on may not be safe to take during pregnancy. Look in your medicine cabinet and note what is safe during pregnancy and what is not. Speak with your doctor if you are not sure. Replace the not-safe-for-pregnancy items with safe options so when a headache does hit, you'll have a proper cure available.

24 Discuss your habits with your doctor to be sure they are safe during pregnancy. There are obvious things to cut out when you find out you're pregnant, like drinking and smoking. Then there are habits that aren't as clear-cut, like if you are caffeine obsessed, love to ski, dye your hair, or enjoy a weekly sushi dinner. Consult your doctor about these habits and learn what is safe and what you'll need to minimize or cut.

• • ♦ • •

25 Keep a cheat sheet of off-limit foods on your phone. There is a long list of foods to avoid when pregnant, and it can be hard to remember each one. For example, some fish is safe while other types should be avoided. Instead of doing an online search every time you are about to eat a new food, save an easy-to-access list recommended by your doctor on your phone. Either keep a running list in a Notes app, or search for a premade graphic from your practice and save it to your phone's favorite images. Make it accessible so you can quickly reference it when ordering at a restaurant or out grocery shopping.

26 **Download a pregnancy app.** Pregnancy apps share interesting, useful, and fun updates, like the recent development of the fetus, symptoms you may be experiencing, and what size fruit or vegetable your baby is each week. Apps may also offer weekly or monthly to-do lists to help you get ready for your baby's arrival.

• • ◆ • •

27 **Sign up for only one or two pregnancy and parenting newsletters.** Pregnancy-related newsletters can be really informational, but don't go overboard and bombard your inbox with dozens of them; choose one or two that you like best. These are a good source of pregnancy and baby information, as well as product recommendations. Some newsletters may offer discounts and samples for pregnancy and newborn products.

28 Take one belly picture each week. Make sure you document the amazing changes your body is experiencing. Even if you don't feel good, are not in the mood for photos, or don't plan to share your bump pictures with the world, chances are, in hindsight, you'll be happy you took them. Start taking bump pictures before you even begin showing so you can really capture the full transformation. To best display your belly growth over the nine months, aim to take a picture each week on the same day and in the exact same spot, keep the background clean, stand in the same pose, and wear the same or similar clothes in each one. Ask your partner to take these for you or set up a tripod and capture it yourself.

••♦••

29 Start a baby name list now and update it frequently. Deciding on a name for your baby can be a challenging task with a lot of pressure attached. Start the brainstorming early! Keep an ongoing list in your phone. Whenever you think of a name that you love or even just like, jot it down. The "maybe" names might spark a new idea that you end up loving. Have your partner start their own list, and every so often cross-reference to see if you have any matching front-runners.

30 **Set an alarm to remember your vitamins.** Set an alarm on your phone or on your smartwatch at the same time each day as a reminder to take your prenatal vitamin. Ideally, you've been taking your vitamin since before getting pregnant, but if not, now is the time to make it a part of your daily routine.

• • ♦ • •

31 **Create a water-drinking schedule to be sure you stay hydrated.** Hydration is very important because being dehydrated can cause complications in pregnancy. Be aware of your water intake, especially in the first trimester, as dehydration caused by morning sickness and vomiting might occur. Establish a daily ounce goal and then break it up into a schedule that's easy to follow. For example, if your goal is 80 ounces per day, aim to drink 20 ounces by 10 a.m., 40 ounces by noon, 60 ounces by 2 p.m., and 80 ounces by 4 p.m. You can even make a daily checklist that you can mark off as you finish each ounce goal or get a special bottle to keep yourself motivated.

32 Calculate your actual caffeine intake in a twenty-four-hour period. Caffeine usually isn't completely off-limits during pregnancy, but it is recommended that you stay under 200 milligrams per day. Decide how much you feel comfortable consuming, then figure out how much you're consuming now (many people don't even know for sure!). Remember, things beyond your morning cup of coffee contain caffeine, like sodas, some teas, and chocolate. Also, there can be a wide range of caffeine content in coffee. A coffee at home, at Starbucks, and at Dunkin' all contain different quantities of caffeine. Make an approximate calculation of how much caffeine you're consuming and cut out certain items or replace some with decaf varieties as needed.

••♦••

33 Pack a plastic bag for on-the-go nausea moments. Always have a plastic bag or two in your purse or car. Nausea can hit at any time, not just in the morning, and not necessarily when you have easy access to a bathroom or trash can. You never know when you may need that plastic bag, and you will be thankful if/when that time comes.

Ideas for Concealing Your Pregnancy at Work

Hiding your pregnancy from coworkers you see every day, for many hours a day, is certainly a challenge. If your energy is low and your pants are bursting at the seams, here are some sneaky ways to keep your pregnancy under wraps in the office.

Start a water challenge with coworkers. Fluctuating hormones and drinking more water can cause you to pee more. If coworkers are suspicious, tell them you're doing a hydration challenge, aiming to drink 100 ounces of water a day. Encourage them to join you. Now you'll all be running to the bathroom between meetings! Note: If you are experiencing morning sickness and are spending a lot of time in the bathroom throwing up, you may want to skip this idea.

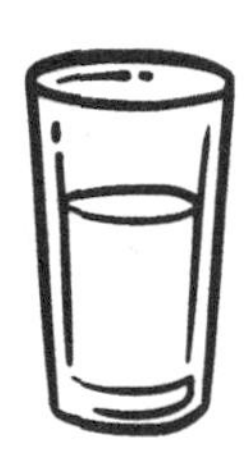

35 **Throw up in a hidden or less-trafficked bathroom.** Trying to hide your pregnancy while throwing up all day? Scope out the bathroom situation in your office building so you don't get stuck trying to throw up in silence while another coworker is mere feet away. Consider a secluded bathroom that's out of the way, a bathroom on a different floor, or even a nearby public restroom.

36 **Claim dental work when going to the ob-gyn.** If you need to go to several doctor's appointments before sharing your news, say you're going to the dentist. It's a believable fib. Most people go to the dentist a couple of times a year, and follow-up visits for cavities, crowns, or other services are common.

37 **Keep crackers at your desk.** If you are experiencing nausea throughout the day, be prepared by keeping bland crackers or whatever snack you prefer in your desk. You can grab these for a quick and discreet bite to soothe your stomach.

38 **Request that meetings start after 11 a.m. if you feel sick in the mornings.** If you're experiencing morning sickness or first trimester exhaustion, avoid scheduling early-morning meetings. Aim for after 11 a.m. if possible.

39 **Claim you are renovating your house and need to work from home.** Working from home isn't an option for everyone, but if it is for you, take it. If you're not feeling great or need alone time, work from home. Say you're having construction done on your house that you need to oversee.

40 **Switch from in-person to video conference calls.** Instead of traveling to in-person meetings, request phone or video chats. If on video, keep the camera aimed at your shoulders and above to avoid any growing belly shots.

41 **Pack lunch and say you're trying to save money.** If your coworkers are often heading out for lunch where it might become obvious that you're pregnant (for example, if you love your weekly sushi outings), bring a homemade lunch and claim that you're on a budget.

42 **Be mindful of your hands and keep them at your sides.** You know how pregnant women are always pictured with their hands on their bellies? There is just something about that growing belly that makes you want to touch it more often than you used to. This is an easy giveaway for suspicious coworkers. Keep this in mind and keep your hands at your sides.

43 **Use a tote bag or other prop to hide your belly.** Thankfully, large tote bags are pretty much always in style. Hold one in front of you or place it in your lap while seated to conceal your belly.

44 **Choose outfits full of patterns and colors.** Big and bold patterns and colors will help camouflage your changing body shape.

45 **Add layers to your outfit.** Select multiple layers when getting dressed. The more flowing layers you have, the more hidden your belly will be.

46 **Cozy up with a blanket scarf to hide your belly.** A big scarf will keep you warm and hide your expanding waistline. The bigger the better! Large scarves will also come in handy as a stylish nursing cover once the baby arrives.

47 **Try a bold lip as a distraction.** Anything to keep prying eyes from your growing belly, right?

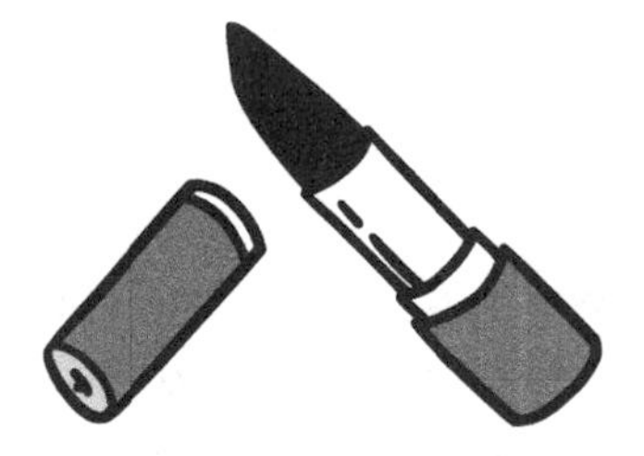

48 Switch to wireless bras to ease breast soreness. One of the first signs of pregnancy may be swollen and tender breasts. Now is a good time to switch to a supportive yet soft and comfortable bra. Choose a wireless style and one that has soft and stretchy cups that can grow with you over the next few months.

••♦••

49 Set a bedtime alarm. Proper sleep is always important, but it is especially vital during pregnancy. Establish a good sleep routine that you can aim to stick with for the rest of your pregnancy. Setting alarms isn't just for waking you up in the morning—you can also set an alarm that signals it is time to get ready for bed.

••♦••

50 Take power naps. First trimester exhaustion is the real deal. Don't fight it—give in and add naps to your schedule. This might be hard if you work at an office, so if you work a nine-to-five job, take a quick nap when you get home. If you find that afternoon naps are making it harder for you to fall asleep at night, consider skipping them. Take advantage of nap opportunities on the weekend in order to feel extra refreshed when Monday rolls around again.

51 Do a one-minute stretch at the top of each hour to refresh yourself. It can be hard to stay active, especially in the early days when you'd prefer to camp out in bed or when you're sitting at a desk most days. Stretching can help keep your energy levels up and can make your body less achy. If you're always forgetting to stretch or can't seem to find the time, try this hack: At the top of each hour, set a timer for sixty seconds and do a few gentle stretches. If you'd prefer to save your stretching for when you're at home, do it while watching TV.

••◆••

52 Reassess your workouts to be sure they're safe. In most cases, there is no reason to stop attending your much-loved group fitness classes or going out for your daily run. Still, check with your doctor as you navigate your fitness routine. Complications or not, there are some adjustments your doctor might recommend. Work with your doctor to set realistic goals while still challenging yourself. Above all, listen to your body.

53 Communicate with your fitness instructor. When attending group fitness classes, tell your instructor that you are pregnant so they can advise you on any changes you should make to the workout. If you don't feel ready to share the news with your instructor, instead say that you are working through some "injuries" and may modify some of the moves in class.

••♦••

54 Consider making friends with other pregnant women in your workout classes. If you happen to spot pregnant women in your classes, take notice. You may learn some modifying techniques to use during class; plus once you're ready to share your pregnancy news, you can make a new friend.

••♦••

55 Use the "talk test" to assess if you are working out too hard. The "talk test" is a simple way to guide your workout intensity during pregnancy. While working out, see if you can comfortably talk and maintain a conversation. If you are panting and struggling to speak a full sentence, this is a warning that you may need to take your intensity down a notch.

56 Switch to grocery delivery to save time and energy. During these exhausting early days, look for small shortcuts that can make your life easier. Avoid unnecessary trips to the grocery store and instead have your groceries delivered. Not to mention, if you are feeling sensitive to smells during the first trimester, the grocery store can be an overwhelming and nausea-inducing place.

• • ♦ • •

57 Confide in one mom friend early on. It can be hard to keep your pregnancy a secret, especially during the first few weeks and months when your mind is in overdrive, processing all the questions you have. Plus, you may be feeling miserable, and it can be helpful to vent to someone who has been there. If you feel comfortable, pick one trustworthy friend to confide in, ideally someone who has also been pregnant. They can be your go-to source for your first trimester pregnancy questions. They can also help steer other friends away from asking you questions (like, why aren't you drinking?) when you're out together.

58 If you're expecting multiples, join an online support group for more specific advice. Twins, triplets, and other multiples make for different types of pregnancies. An online forum can give you important information and suggestions about multiples pregnancy, labor and delivery, and parenting.

•• ♦ ••

59 Plan ahead on how you'll announce your news. Some people announce their pregnancy as soon as they get a positive test, while others wait until the second trimester or longer. Align with your partner on when to announce the news. If you're telling family before others, make sure they are also aware of when you are going public with the news so they don't spoil the surprise. Once you've decided, plan your announcement in a way that matches your personality and interests. Get creative and use a letterboard, dress up your dogs as they prepare for their new sibling, time the announcement around a holiday and use themed props, or just keep it simple and share the news.

PARTNER HACKS

How to Make the First Trimester Go Smoothly

60 **Prepare bland meals, light on seasoning.** Now probably isn't the time to get creative in the kitchen—wait until you see what cravings appear. Until then, keep things super simple and light on seasonings. If your partner is experiencing nausea, bland foods may help soothe her symptoms. Stick to those bland foods for yourself as well; your nauseous partner probably isn't interested in seeing or smelling your more adventurous meal.

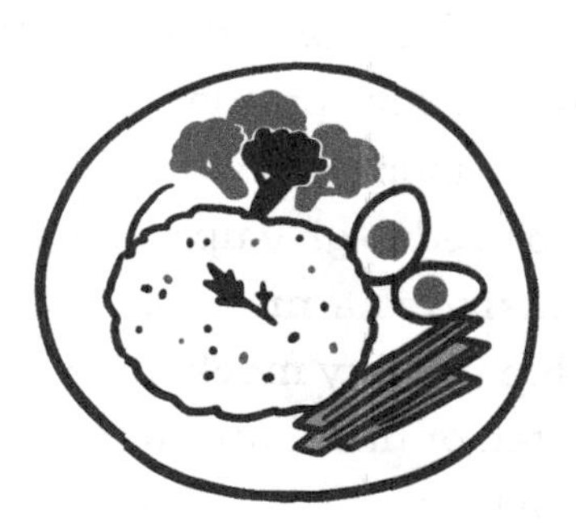

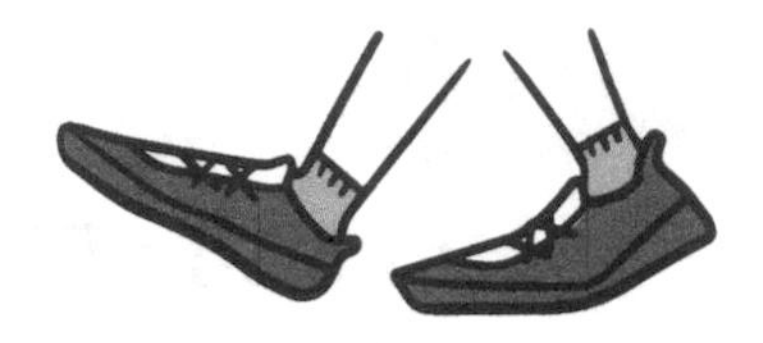

61 **Cut down on caffeine and suggest morning or evening walks.** Being healthy shouldn't just fall on the shoulders of your partner! Now is a good time to make your entire household a healthier place. By adopting healthy habits of your own, you can support and positively impact your partner's actions as well. If she drops her caffeine consumption, do the same. And if you're both trying to stay more active, suggest a morning or evening walk each day as a time to get in some steps while connecting with each other.

62 **Switch to seltzer and don't drink alcohol out of solidarity.** Your partner won't be drinking for quite a few months, and while technically you don't also need to give up alcohol, taking a break from drinking is a nice way to show your support. Whip up tasty mocktails, stock up on sparkling water, or blend up smoothies that you can enjoy together.

63 **Do a big grocery haul and make sure the pantry is always stocked with snacks.** Your partner's appetite might be all over the map at first, so be ready for anything. Keep your pantry well stocked with her favorite items, specifically making sure she has plenty of the few foods she can stomach during the first trimester when she may be pickier than normal.

64 **Create a list of chores that you will do instead of your partner.** Now is the time to step up your chore game. Don't wait for your exhausted partner to ask you to do a load of laundry or vacuum the rug. Just go ahead and do it. To stay on top of it, write down a list of things you will do and your partner should skip. Update as necessary as the weeks go by.

65 **Keep her glass filled with water at all times.** Staying hydrated is important throughout all stages of pregnancy, and the first trimester is a great time to get into this habit. Help your partner by always keeping her water bottle or glass filled and encouraging her to continue sipping.

66 **Maintain a clean bathroom.** If your partner is constantly heading to the bathroom to vomit, the last thing she'll want when she gets there is to discover that it's a mess. Make it your mission to keep the bathroom sparkling clean, especially the floor and toilet.

67 **Change the sheets so your partner can rest well.** Your partner may experience an increase in sweating while pregnant. Waking up in sweaty sheets isn't a great feeling, and a simple yet much-appreciated task for you to handle is to change and clean the sheets on a regular basis.

68 **Keep your physical complaints to yourself.** Whatever ache or pain you might be feeling, keep it to yourself. Tired from a long day at work? Keep that to yourself as well. Your pregnant partner is probably feeling more aches and pains and is more tired, so vent to a friend instead.

69 **Attend doctor's appointments.** You aren't required to be at all the appointments, but remember that you're in this together. If you can make it to prenatal appointments with your partner, you'll feel more involved and your partner will feel more supported. Come prepared with any questions you have; this will show your partner that you are excited and invested.

70 **Ask your partner how she is feeling.** Your partner may be the one carrying the baby, but you can stay involved and learn more by asking questions about how she is feeling. Check in frequently and do what you can to keep her comfortable.

71 **Speak with HR and explore your parental leave.** Start looking into what is offered at your office, and begin to figure out what life will look like once the baby arrives.

CHAPTER 2

Making Your Wardrobe Work

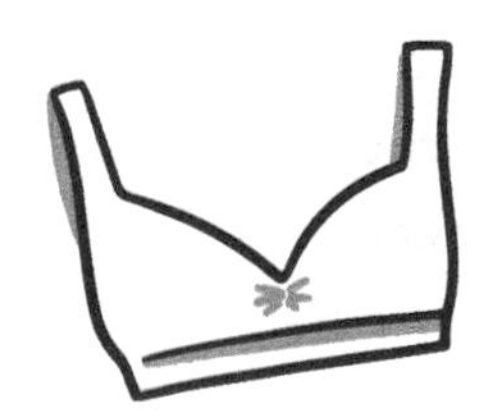

Now that your body is constantly changing, your wardrobe will also need to undergo a transformation. Whether your bump is making its first appearance or you're already struggling to button your jeans, this chapter will give you fashion hacks to make getting dressed in the morning a simple task. This chapter has all your clothing questions covered, including ways to maximize how long you can wear your current wardrobe, creative solutions to make your wardrobe seem larger if you're on a budget, plus recommendations for the best items to add to your maternity closet. In short—you'll find everything you need to feel comfortable and confident throughout your pregnancy.

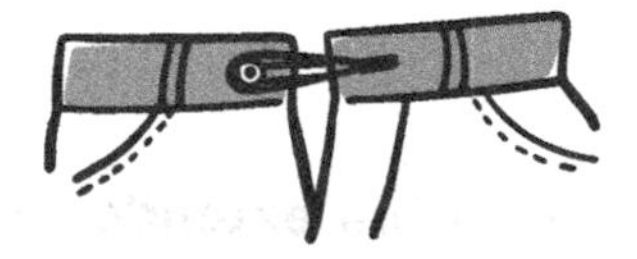

72 Use hair elastics to extend your waistbands. Hair ties can make your pre-pregnancy jeans last as long as possible before you switch over to maternity jeans. Thread a hair elastic through the buttonhole of your jeans, then loop the hairband back over the button to secure your pants. Wear with a tunic or long shirt to ensure the zipper, hair tie, and button stay hidden.

• • ♦ • •

73 Buy bra extenders to keep wearing your pre-pregnancy bras. Bra extenders are extra hooks that are easily added to your current bras. These will extend the band of your bras so you can continue with your current stash, even as your rib cage expands. A pack of extenders typically costs less than $10—far less expensive than new bras.

74 Make your own bra extender with an old bra. You can even make your own bra extender. All you need is an old bra you're willing to part with and a needle and thread. Cut the hook-and-eye portion off the old bra, then sew the old portion onto a current bra's hook-and-eye portion. Ta-da, you've added extra inches to your current bra! Look online for how-to details and photos to follow.

• • ♦ • •

75 Buy a belly band so you can keep wearing pre-pregnancy pants and tops. Belly bands are large, looped pieces of stretchy fabric that will allow you to keep wearing your pre-pregnancy pants and tops. Position the belly band right at your waistband, and it will help to keep your unbuttoned pants up and your belly covered (if your shirt rides up because it's getting too short).

76 Make your own belly band out of a tank top. Save some money and make your own. Simply cut a stretchy tank top in half. (The more stretchy and supportive the material, the better—tank tops made with spandex work well.) After the material is cut, simply position it at your pant line to smooth out your waistline. Sew the edge if the tank top material is fraying.

• • ♦ • •

77 Wear a tank top as a bra. If you made a belly band from the bottom of a tank top, don't toss the top of it. If the material is tight and stretchy enough, you can wear it as a comfortable bra for lounging around your house (it won't be particularly supportive, but with sore and sensitive breasts common in pregnancy, light support like this may be just what you want).

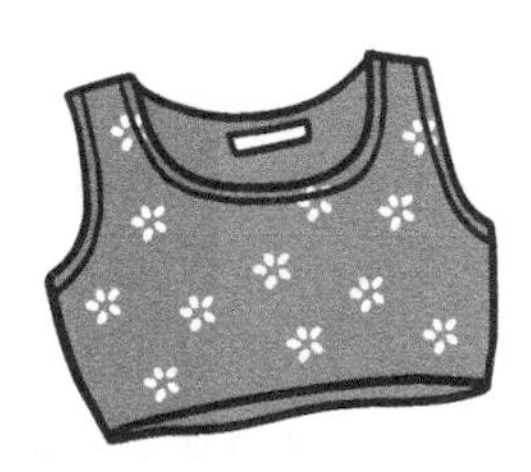

78 Buy bigger bras if necessary, but don't buy nursing bras yet. It is tempting to buy items in preparation for after the baby arrives, but hold off on purchasing nursing bras if you plan to breastfeed. During pregnancy your boobs have probably grown, and it might seem impossible that they will get any larger—but once your milk comes in, there is a good chance that they will indeed get bigger. If you buy nursing bras for your current (pregnant) size, they may not fit by the time you're breastfeeding.

• • ♦ • •

79 Keep wearing your pre-pregnancy jacket with the addition of a jacket extender. Pregnant in the winter? You'll only be able to zip up your coat for so long unless you buy a jacket extender. Jacket extenders zipper an extra panel of fabric into your current jacket's zipper, giving it extra room. These can be somewhat pricey, but they're probably cheaper than buying a maternity coat, and once the baby arrives, you continue using it—if you wear your baby in a carrier, the jacket can cozily zip around both of you.

80 Make your own jacket extender with a piece of fabric. Own a sewing machine and prefer to make your own jacket extender? Find patterns to follow online and create your own jacket extender to use this winter. You don't need a lot of materials—typically just a piece of fabric, two zippers, and thread. Look for fabric that is a close match to your jacket, so the extender will seamlessly blend in.

••◆••

81 Buy new shoes a half or one size larger than your current shoe size. Along with all the other things growing bigger, your feet may grow during pregnancy. The size change can be temporary due to swelling, or your feet may stay at the larger size for the long haul. If your shoes are feeling snug, purchase a pair the next size up to keep yourself comfortable.

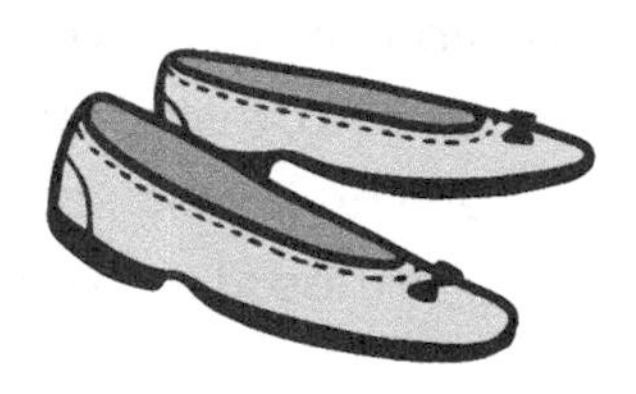

82 Look in the back of your closet for old clothes that may get a second chance with your new body. Before you make your first maternity purchase, take a trip into your closet and look at things with new eyes. Are there items that are not maternity-specific but might be useful? That baggy sweater that you never wear because you thought it was unflattering might be the perfect item to dress your bump. Or maybe you have a pair of stretched-out jeans that you stopped wearing a while ago. As you go through your closet, think of things in terms of your new body, and you might find some hidden gems that deserve a second life.

• • ♦ • •

83 Create slip-on shoes by adding elastic laces. Eventually, it's going to become a challenge to bend over and tie your shoes. You don't have to buy something new, though—just take your current sneakers and turn them into slip-ons: Remove the current lacing. Replace the laces with thinly cut elastic cord, a thin bungee cord, or elastic shoelaces. Tie off the ends in a way that allows the shoes to slip on your feet and stay there.

84 Slip on compression socks to combat swelling. Mild swelling in the feet and ankles is normal during pregnancy. Compression socks may reduce swelling. Find compression socks that feel firm and tight, but not to an uncomfortable degree. Put them on in the morning, as they may keep swelling from getting worse throughout the day. If you're an athlete, hang on to your compression socks for after pregnancy. You can wear them after intense workouts to aid in muscle recovery.

••◆••

85 Buy maternity items a few at a time. There are some pretty cute maternity clothes on the market, so it can be tempting to buy a whole wardrobe worth of new items as soon as your bump appears. Slow down. Your body is going to go through a lot of changes. What fits perfectly one week is suddenly too tight the next week. Only buy a couple of items at a time and continue to shop as your body and your needs change.

Must-Have Maternity Wear

A totally new wardrobe isn't necessary during pregnancy, but the addition of a few key items will ensure you stay comfortable and confident during your pregnancy. Here are some items worth adding to your current wardrobe.

86 **A flattering blazer that will make you feel professional and stylish.** For a chic and easy-to-wear work-appropriate outfit, add a blazer. Since they are typically worn open, it will continue to fit, even as your belly continues to grow (and after the baby has arrived!).

87 **Button-down shirts that will work during and after pregnancy.** Quality button-downs can last the length of pregnancy, and even beyond. During the smaller bump stages, wear the shirt buttoned. As your belly grows, you can continue to wear these tops unbuttoned, layered over a stretchy tank top. And finally, if the sizing works out, button-down shirts are a great choice for nursing.

88 **A trendy belt to add shape to clothes.** Want to add shape to a larger maternity dress or top? Simply add a belt above your belly.

89 **An always-in-style wrap coat to eliminate zippers and buttons.** If you don't want to deal with jacket extenders or a too-small coat, instead buy a chic wrap coat. Purchase a size larger than normal so it can easily accommodate your growing belly.

90 **One good pair of maternity jeans that you feel great in.** There's no need to go overboard with a large collection of maternity jeans that you will only wear for a few months. Focus on one quality pair that has a good stretch panel, allowing you to wear them throughout pregnancy. Some styles have a stretch panel that goes all the way over your bump, and others have side paneling that stretches at your sides. Try on a variety of styles and see what fits and flatters your body and bump type. Do some squats and lunges, and walk around as you try on styles. See what stays in place, doesn't slip down your bump, and what you feel most comfortable in.

91 **Well-fitting underwear.** A relatively low-cost upgrade, new underwear is a simple pleasure in life that, as a pregnant woman, you deserve. As your body size and shape change during pregnancy, give your underwear drawer a nice refresh and feel like a new woman.

92 **A large tote bag or backpack to carry all your necessities.** A good bag will come in handy throughout pregnancy. You may find that you're carrying more gear than you typically would, like a large water bottle, snacks, and so on. A large tote bag will do the trick. If a tote bag is throwing off your balance or hurting your back, switch to a supportive backpack that has soft straps to alleviate shoulder pain.

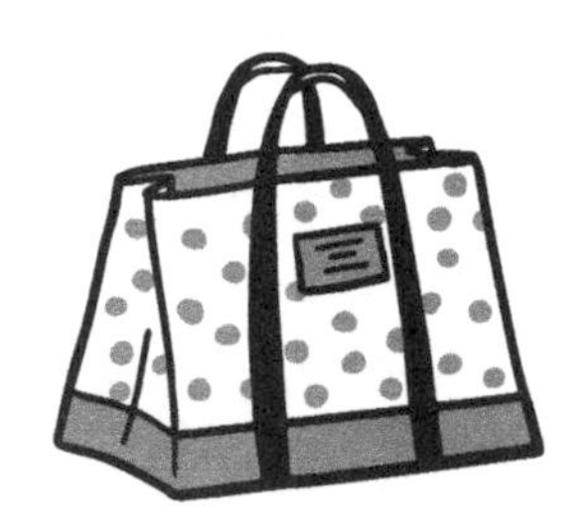

93 **Versatile flats for comfortable and supportive walking.** If you love wearing heels and want to keep that as a part of your wardrobe, go for it. For many women, though, pregnancy is a time to focus on comfort. (Not to mention, wearing heels during pregnancy can put extra pressure on your back, knees, and ankle joints.) It also may be a safer choice to switch to flats, as pregnancy can impact your balance. Find a pair of high-quality flats that you love.

94 **High-waisted leggings with good stretch for lounging.** There are plenty of maternity leggings to choose from, but once you give birth, these will quickly no longer fit, giving them a pretty short life span. Instead of only buying maternity-specific leggings, look for nonmaternity, high-waisted leggings. (The higher the waist, the better.) If you opt for a higher-quality legging, the high-waisted portion won't permanently stretch out and can then be used postpartum. High-waisted leggings are an excellent way to stay covered while breastfeeding as well.

95 **Supportive and breathable sandals for the hottest days.** If you are pregnant during summer months, a good pair of sandals is a must. They allow extra room for swelling, keep your feet cool, and usually don't require bending over to put them on (slip-ons are ideal!). Select a pair that are structured and provide balance and support.

96 **Supportive bras to accommodate your growing chest.** Your bra size may change drastically throughout pregnancy. Once your current bras (or bra extenders) are no longer serving you, shop for a handful of new bras that are comfortable and supportive.

97 **Workout clothes you love and will love to work out in.** Thanks to stretchy material, you'll be able to wear workout gear longer than your more structured and constricting items (goodbye, jeans!). Also, if you like your workout clothes, you may be more inclined to work out and may even feel more confident during your time at the gym. Staying active throughout pregnancy can make you feel better and stronger as you approach your due date.

98 Shop during your second trimester for postpartum items. Once you hit your second trimester, you can start thinking ahead to your first few months with the baby. What will the weather be like, and what will you want to wear? If you're planning to breastfeed, you'll need nursing-friendly clothes. The first few months after childbirth, your body will be around the same size it is in the second trimester. When buying tops to wear during the second trimester, consider nursing tank tops with strap clips, and flowy tops that will work well for both pregnancy and nursing.

• • ◆ • •

99 Shop at secondhand shops for discounted good-quality maternity wear. With a quickly changing body, it's no wonder that maternity clothes stay in good shape; you usually only wear them for a few months. That's why shopping secondhand is a great way to stock up on maternity wear. It's less expensive than buying new, and items are typically in good condition. Check local secondhand shops or online thrift sites. Oftentimes secondhand children's stores will have a maternity section. And once you're done with your maternity wear, resell it and recoup some of that cost.

100 Purchase items made from stretchy material for clothes that will fit for multiple months. Stretchy dresses and tops made of cotton jersey and spandex are a great choice for pregnancy. They will continue to stretch as your belly grows, and they are also a comfortable option for the postpartum period. When you try on clothes, give items a tug to ensure that they will not become see-through as your belly and body expand.

••♦••

101 Use a clothing rental service for special occasions. Attending a wedding or special event while pregnant? Shopping for an outfit can be frustrating and can feel like a waste of money if you will only wear it once. Instead of buying, rent maternity wear for big occasions. This saves money and is less environmentally wasteful.

102 Sign up for a maternity rental subscription and let someone else do the shopping for you. If getting to the store is a challenge with your schedule, sign up for a maternity clothes subscription or rental box. Some companies offer monthly shipments that are curated with your stage of pregnancy in mind, while others allow you to select specific items, wear them for a certain amount of time, then send them back in exchange for new items. These services take the guesswork and effort out of finding clothes that fit your ever-changing body.

• • ♦ • •

103 Shop your friends' closets for their old maternity wear. If you have friends who have kids and aren't currently pregnant, ask to take a shopping trip through their closet. Chances are that they have some maternity wear shoved in the back that isn't getting any use right now. Ask your friends who were pregnant during the same seasons you are, in order to find weather-appropriate items.

104 Buy a hat you love to protect yourself from the sun. During pregnancy, some women experience melasma, or what some refer to as the "mask of pregnancy," a condition where parts of your skin (usually on your face) can turn brown or grayish. This may be caused or exacerbated by sun exposure. If you're prone to melasma, find a stylish hat that you don't mind wearing, and your skin will thank you.

• • ♦ • •

105 Switch to online shopping to avoid uncomfortable and small dressing rooms. If entering a tiny changing room with your belly is an anxiety-inducing activity, do your shopping online. Use sites that offer free shipping and free returns. Don't be afraid to try multiple sizes and styles so you can see what works best. Your body size is totally new, and finding things that fit and that you feel good in is a new challenge. When your package arrives, make note of how you feel. If you are not in the mood for a try-on session, leave it for later, or you may end up not liking anything. Try on the clothes when you're in a good mood and send back whatever doesn't serve you.

106 Create a capsule collection to more easily get dressed in the morning. To minimize the hassle of getting dressed in the morning, find a handful of maternity items that you love and feel good in. This capsule collection will be a small group of simple items that you can rotate and re-wear in different combinations. If wearing the same thing for your entire pregnancy doesn't appeal to you, re-create your capsule collection on a monthly basis. Keep some basic items that work well, but swap in new layering pieces, accessories, and so on.

••◆••

107 Rock your bikini instead of buying a new one-piece. Don't be afraid to show off that growing bump! If you're heading to the pool or beach while pregnant, you can skip buying maternity-specific bathing suits and instead wear two-pieces that you already own. These are actually more likely to fit than a non-maternity one-piece and can get you through a good portion of your pregnancy.

108 Embrace the bump with formfitting clothing. If your first trimester was spent hiding your bump, when the news is out, you might want to embrace that growing belly. Showing off your bump with fitted clothing can often be more flattering than oversized and shapeless styles.

••◆••

109 Focus on accessories. Love to shop but aren't a fan of maternity wear and its typically short life span? Upgrade your accessories. Dress up a simple maternity outfit with a new bag, jewelry, sunglasses, or headband that you absolutely love. This is a great idea if you are feeling frustrated with maternity clothes—instead embrace accessories that you can continue to use.

••◆••

110 Wear breathable fabrics, especially in the summer. You may sweat more while pregnant, so stick to breathable fabrics like lightweight cotton, linen, and other natural fibers that are typically better at soaking up moisture from the skin. Avoid nylon, silk, and polyester on particularly hot days.

111 Cover your belly button with adhesive bandages. At a certain point in pregnancy, your belly button is likely to stick out. It's not a big deal, but if you're wearing a silk top or are dressed up and would prefer not to have your belly button visible, cover it with a nipple cover or an adhesive bandage. This is also a good solution if your belly button is uncomfortably rubbing against your clothes.

••◆••

112 Use Windex to remove rings that are stuck on. Rings won't budge off your swollen hands? Don't panic. Soak your finger in Windex or soap and water, and then try to loosen the ring and slide it off your hand.

••◆••

113 Take your rings off at the first signs of hand swelling. If you're experiencing swelling in your hands, there may come a day when it's too hard to get your rings off. Take note of hand swelling and stop wearing your rings before it becomes too painful to remove them.

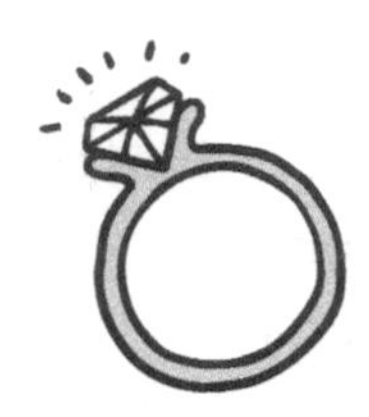

114 Try dental floss for really stuck-on rings. If wetting your hand didn't help, grab about 12 inches of dental floss and thread it under your ring, and then wind the floss around your finger again and again, up to your knuckle. This process should gently compress your swollen finger. Now take the end of the string that is under the ring and unwrap the floss, quickly trying to get the ring over your knuckle and off your finger.

••◆••

115 Wear your rings as a necklace or get a fake ring. If you don't want to part with your engagement ring and wedding band for the remainder of your pregnancy, wear it on a very sturdy chain around your neck, or purchase a faux diamond ring in a larger ring size that you can wear on your hand instead.

PARTNER HACKS

How to Help with Her Clothes

116 **Give her free rein of your closet.** If you are larger than your partner, go ahead and share your closet. She may find some items that make her feel extra comfy and cozy at home, like sweatshirts, oversized T-shirts, button-downs, or even your winter coat if she's running out for a quick walk around the block.

117 **Tie her shoes.** One day during pregnancy, your partner will suddenly lose sight of her feet and tying her shoes will be a big challenge. Don't just watch the struggle; get down there and tie her shoes for her.

118 **Get a bag or backpack to carry her things.** Pregnant women may need a few extra things when they leave the house (it's always a good idea to pack water and a snack!). Offer to carry her bag, and if her bag is not your style, invest in a nice unisex tote bag or backpack that you won't mind toting around.

119 **Go shopping with her.** Join your partner for her shopping trips. It's another easy way for you to support her and be involved.

120 **Expect some costs for new clothes.** As your partner's wearable wardrobe dwindles while her belly grows, she'll need to spend money to purchase new items that fit and that she feels good in. Get on the same page about a budget that fits your financial situation, but be understanding that she will need some new items.

121 **Buy her a special gift.** Now is a nice time to get your partner something meaningful. Maybe it's a splurge-worthy pair of maternity jeans that she'll feel great wearing, or an accessory that will bring her some joy.

122 **Tell your partner that she looks good.** Through all of this, your job is to remain your partner's biggest and most loyal cheerleader. At times she may feel physically uncomfortable as her body changes; your job is to reassure her that she is beautiful and that you love her through all the amazing changes.

CHAPTER 3

Keeping Your Body Feeling Good

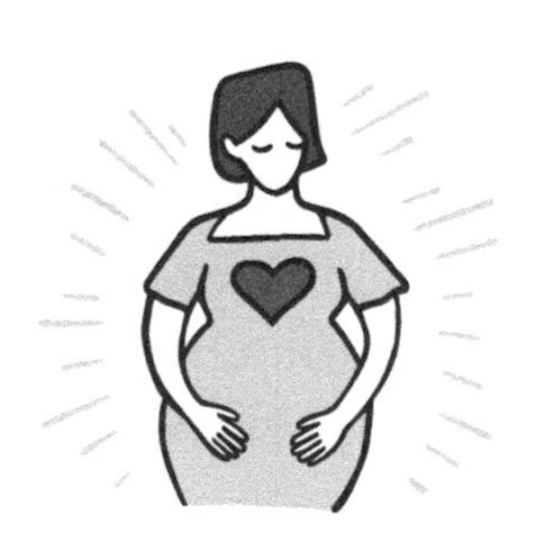

It's amazing what your body is capable of, and during pregnancy you'll have a front-row seat to the incredible evolution. Just when you think your belly couldn't possibly get any bigger to support the baby's growth, somehow it does. Along with the incredible and beautiful moments, there will no doubt be common aches and pains to deal with as well. This chapter will offer dozens of suggestions for relieving, avoiding, or at least minimizing these annoyances.

Every woman's experience is totally unique. Some women never experience morning sickness, some only in the first trimester, and others feel ill all nine months. There are other things you may or may not experience as well, like stretch marks and back pain. And though there isn't a tried-and-true magic potion to help everyone eliminate stretch marks or avoid back pain, there are plenty of tactics to try. Hopefully some of these ideas will give you much-desired relief. Read on for hacks to battle morning sickness, dry and tight skin, sore muscles, and more.

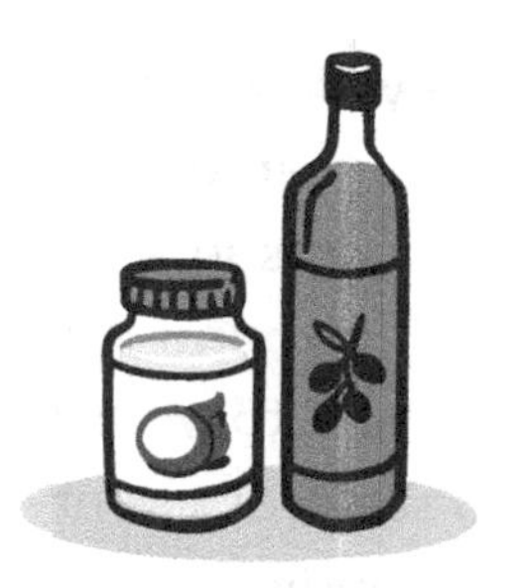

123 Use cooking oils to soothe itchy skin. If you're experiencing tight, itchy, and dry skin, particularly on your belly, look in your kitchen for a solution, not your medicine cabinet. Rub olive oil or coconut oil onto your belly for moisturizing relief.

••◆••

124 Keep skin hydrated with pregnancy-safe body butter. If you'd prefer to keep your body care separate from your pantry staples, buy body oil or belly butter to use on your belly, hips, and thighs. Some believe that a good moisturizing routine can help with stretch marks, while others say it is genetics. Either way, staying moisturized will keep your skin feeling soft and smooth. Seek out brands that offer pregnancy-specific body lotions to avoid harmful chemicals.

125 Reduce itchy skin with a soothing oatmeal bath. An oatmeal bath can do wonders for dry, itchy skin. Simply grind up oats in a blender until smooth. Add ¼ cup of finely ground oats to a warm bath (match the temperature to your body temp, around 98.6°F or less) and soak for twenty minutes. The oatmeal can help your body hold in moisture and may reduce itching.

• • ♦ • •

126 Use a baby bath thermometer to check your water temperature. Did you register for a cute baby bath thermometer toy? Open it up early and use it for your own bath to ensure your bathwater is not too hot. Bathwater above 98.6°F may raise your body temperature, which can be dangerous during pregnancy.

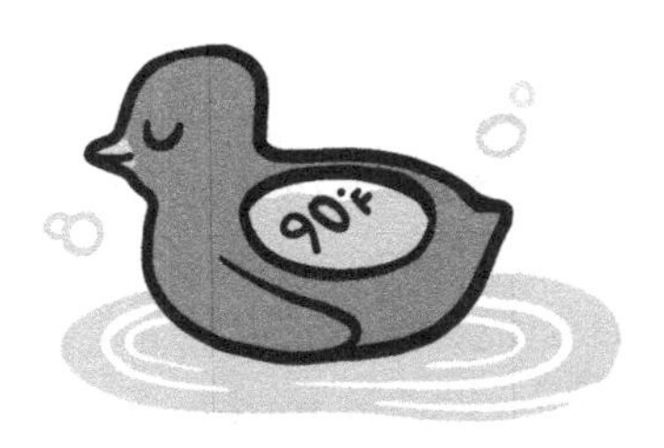

127 Add a scoop of collagen powder to your morning coffee or tea for skin and protein benefits. Collagen supplements may help support skin health, which in turn may help you avoid stretch marks. Research on the topic is mixed, so discuss with your doctor if this idea might be right for you. Collagen also provides a great protein boost, and sufficient protein is important for maintaining balanced nutrition during pregnancy.

••◆••

128 Sprinkle cornstarch in your bra to avoid boob sweat. With potentially increased sweating and fuller breasts during pregnancy, boob sweat is a real thing you might be battling. Cornstarch is absorbent and can pull sweat away from the skin, eliminating sweat that might drip through your bra and onto your shirt. (If you'd prefer to get fancier than cornstarch, there are products available specifically formulated to fight boob sweat.)

129 **Absorb sweat with an ultra-thin panty liner in your bra.** And if you're really sweating through your bras and shirts, panty liners might be the solution. Take a thin panty liner, cut it as needed to properly fit, and stick it inside your bra where you are finding sweat accumulating. This should soak up any sweat before it escapes to your shirt.

••♦••

130 **Store your bra in the freezer for a cooling sensation when you need it.** This hack is simple but can feel so good! On really hot days, chill your bra in the freezer for a few hours before wearing it. You'll get an extra refreshing cooldown when you put it on.

••♦••

131 **Grab long-handled kitchen tongs to help pick up things off the floor.** As your body expands, it will become trickier to bend or squat to pick up something on the floor. If this happens to you, use the tongs to help you retrieve whatever you've dropped.

132 **Use gel pads to ease nipple sensitivity.** If you are pregnant during cold weather, you may experience uncomfortable nipple pain and sensitivity due to the low temperatures. Purchase small, round gel pads that can be heated in the microwave. Heat according to directions (make sure they do not get too hot) and then place in your bra, over your nipples, before going outside. If you have a bra that has an insert space for padding, you can place the gel pad into the insert to have light fabric between the gel pad and your nipple. If possible, look for pads that can be both heated and cooled. You can use the frozen version to address breastfeeding nipple soreness if and when the time comes.

• • ♦ • •

133 **Bend at the knees to reduce back strains.** Between your changing size and shifted center of balance, it's important to be aware of your body positioning. Bend at your knees instead of your waist and avoid twisting as you bend.

Ideas for Fighting Heartburn

Heartburn is an uncomfortable feeling that many women experience during pregnancy. Folklore says it means your child will be born with a lot of hair, but more likely it's caused by progesterone, a hormone that relaxes muscles during pregnancy, including the stomach valve that keeps acid out of your esophagus. Plus, the growing uterus taking over your abdomen may lead to acid going into the esophagus. Whatever causes it, heartburn can be a real pain. Here are some tactics that you can employ that may reduce this burning and uncomfortable sensation.

134 **Keep a food diary to understand your heartburn triggers.** Different foods are triggers for different people. Keep a food diary to see what may be impacting your heartburn and cut those foods out of your daily diet. Common culprits are acidic, fatty, and fried foods. Consider passing on tomatoes, onions, citrus fruits, and chocolate, as these foods may make heartburn worse.

135 **Stock your nightstand with heartburn-fighting products.** Heartburn and acid reflux can strike at night, being particularly uncomfortable in the middle of the night when you've been lying down. Keep essentials, like a pregnancy-safe antacid and cold water, within arm's reach at night.

136 **Elevate your head in bed.** When sleeping, it is beneficial to have your head higher than your stomach, which can help prevent stomach acid from coming up into your esophagus. Do this by placing the head of your bed on risers or on a couple of books. If that's unstable, use extra pillows or buy a wedge to fit under the head of your mattress to ensure your head stays elevated.

137 **Eat smaller meals and eat them slowly.** Instead of three square meals a day, spread your meals out into smaller segments, well spaced throughout the day. When you sit down to eat, really take your time. Eat slowly and thoroughly chew your food.

138 **Try papaya enzymes to battle heartburn.** Unripe papaya is on the do-not-eat list during pregnancy, but papaya enzymes are a different case. Papaya enzymes come in a chewable tablet form and can be used to combat heartburn, but check with your doctor first.

139 **Sit or stand after eating.** Avoid lying down directly after eating. This can cause the stomach acid to rise into your esophagus.

140 **Buy a reusable water bottle and keep it filled.** Staying hydrated can help alleviate heartburn. Buy a reusable water bottle that you don't mind lugging around with you everywhere.

141 **Don't eat large meals too close to bedtime.** Since lying down after eating can exacerbate heartburn, try to allow several hours between your last meal and bedtime.

142 **Sleep on your left side.** This sleeping position may reduce heartburn and is also a recommended way to sleep during pregnancy anyway (since it increases the flow of blood and nutrients to the placenta).

143 Practice new Activities of Daily Living for pregnancy and new mom life. Activities of Daily Living are the moves and actions you take in everyday life. Learning pregnancy-related moves now will prepare you with a new set of actions that will become a part of your daily life when you are a mom: Picking up a baby out of the crib, carrying around a heavy car seat, and standing up from a seated position on the ground with a baby in your arms are just a couple of examples. Check out these new moves, learn which muscle groups are used, and make sure you know the proper form so you can avoid injury. (A personal trainer that specializes in pre- and postnatal training can help you learn and practice proper form.)

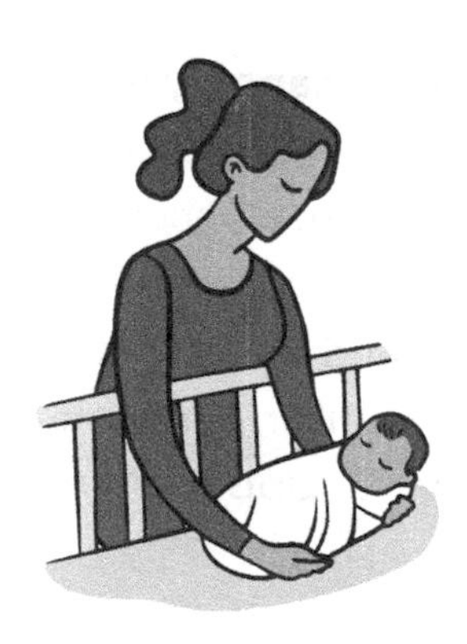

144 Buy a pregnancy pillow to sleep easier at night. Pregnancy is exhausting, but it can be hard to get a good night's sleep. Most doctors recommend that women stop sleeping on their back starting in the second trimester, around twenty weeks, because sleeping on your back can compress the vena cava, a major blood vessel. This can cause nausea, dizziness, and shortness of breath, and can even reduce blood flow to the fetus—plus, it's just plain uncomfortable for most women. A large pregnancy body pillow can offer support to make side sleeping—the ideal sleeping position during pregnancy—more comfortable.

••◆••

145 Make a pregnancy pillow yourself. If you don't want to spend the money on a store-bought pregnancy pillow or are concerned that these giant pillows will take over your bed, make your own. Search for patterns online and find one that fits your needs. You will need fabric, filler, a needle and thread, and, for some patterns, a zipper. A sewing machine is recommended.

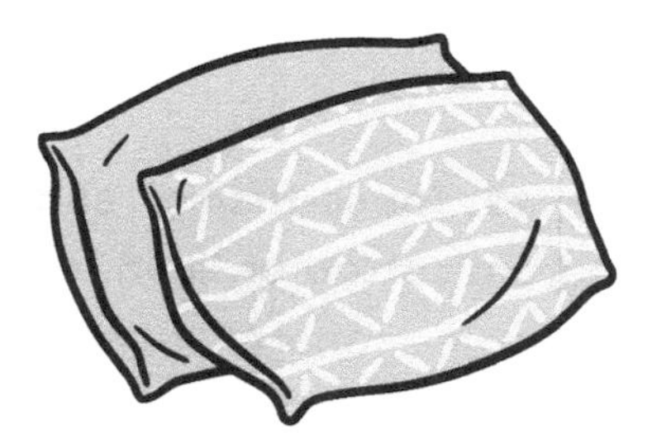

146 Collect the pillows in your home to create a comfortable sleeping position. The easiest route for finding comfort is to simply load up your bed with pillows. Stockpile small throw pillows, your guest pillows, and any extra pillows you can get your hands on—maybe even a couch cushion—near your bed. You can use various sizes to help get your head and back into a good position and grab the smallest ones to help support your bump.

• • ◆ • •

147 Request extra pillows at the concierge when you're staying at a hotel. When you're traveling, call the front desk and request extra pillows. Do this well before bedtime so you don't find yourself awake in the middle of the night wishing you had more support.

148 Switch to loose-fitting and lightweight pajamas made from cotton or linen to combat night sweats. Because of hormonal changes, you may experience night sweats during pregnancy. In most cases, this is nothing to worry about, but it can be uncomfortable. Choose airy pajamas made from moisture-wicking materials. Keep these pajamas handy for postpartum as well, when night sweats might still bother you.

•◆•

149 Track your high- and low-energy times. In your planner or digital calendar, note which hours you feel most energized and productive. Think of these as your "happy hours." No, not *that* kind of happy hour. Figure out what times you feel your best, and do your work or workouts during those hours. Try to spend the hours that you know you are more likely to feel ill in bed resting. By keeping track in a planner, you may start to see a pattern and can better plan your days.

150 Cool down your bedroom before sleeping. Be sure your bedroom isn't too warm at night—setting up a fan could help a lot. A bedroom fan is also great to have once the baby arrives, as bedrooms with fans and rooms that are well ventilated lower a baby's risk of sudden infant death syndrome (SIDS).

• • ✦ • •

151 Wear a smartwatch to ensure you move enough. You might want to consider investing in a smartwatch, like a Fitbit or Apple Watch, to do the work for you. These devices have settings that can vibrate if you haven't taken enough steps within each hour. You can use this well beyond pregnancy as well.

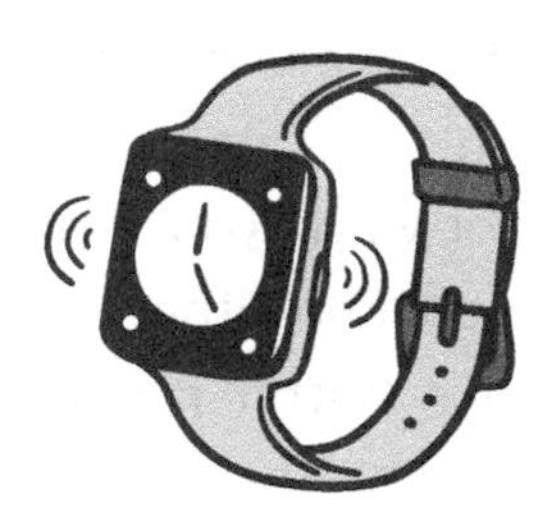

152 Set a timer to go off each hour as a reminder to take a five-minute walk. It's important to try to stay active, even though you may be tired or uncomfortable. Though it may seem counterintuitive, staying active is actually a way to combat many pregnancy aches and discomforts! There is no need to commit to a big workout routine if that's not for you. Even little five-minute walks throughout the day can add up to a more active lifestyle. If you work at a desk and find yourself sitting for many consecutive hours at a time, set a timer to go off every sixty minutes as a signal to get up and move.

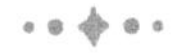

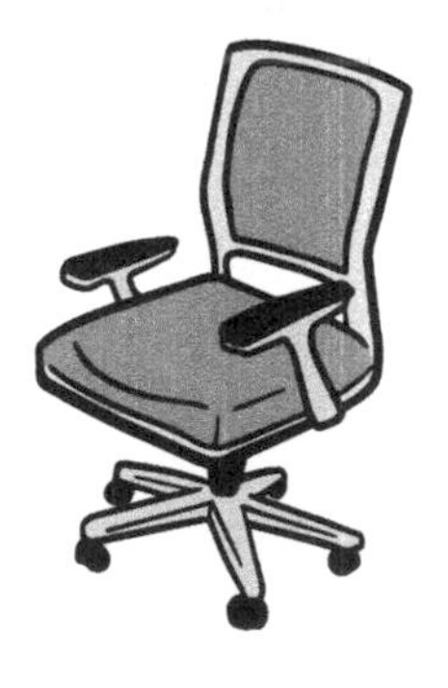

153 Upgrade to an ergonomic chair to promote good posture. If you are experiencing back pain and feel your shoulders slumping forward, you may want to get a new chair that can help you practice better posture, both at work and at home.

154 Apply a cold compress to combat pregnancy-induced carpal tunnel. Pregnant women may be at an increased risk of experiencing carpal tunnel syndrome. If you have numbness, tingling, or throbbing in your hands, wrists, and fingers; swollen fingers; and/or are struggling to grip objects; you may have carpal tunnel syndrome. Speak with your doctor if you are experiencing these issues. Potential solutions include limiting activities that require bending your wrists, elevating your wrists, and using a cold compress on your wrists throughout the day and soft wrist braces at night.

• • ♦ • •

155 Use railings for balance. During pregnancy, you will want to be more mindful of your balance. With a changing body shape and weight, it's no shock that your balance may be impacted. Exercise caution when doing anything that could impact your balance—for example, when working out, try to avoid moves that have you balance on one leg or on uneven surfaces, and use railings or support mechanisms for assistance. Also, be careful when walking on slippery surfaces, uneven sidewalks, or slick stairways—again, look for handrails and use them!

156 Sign up for prenatal Pilates to promote strength during pregnancy and during labor. It's ideal to stay active during pregnancy, so it's worth the effort to find a safe and effective way to move your body. Search for prenatal Pilates classes in your area (or online); it's an activity that can alleviate back pain and may eventually help with labor and delivery.

••◆••

157 Try prenatal yoga for a good stretch, for calming vibes, and to practice breathing and relaxation techniques. Yoga is an amazing way to stay healthy during pregnancy. It's low impact and, with certain modifications, can be done through each trimester of pregnancy. Yoga can promote a calm mind, help with proper breathing patterns, improve your balance, and relieve common pregnancy aches and pains with gentle stretching. Being physically strong during pregnancy is a great way to cultivate a deeper inner strength and resilience. Prenatal-specific classes are also a nice way to connect with other expectant mothers.

158 Do Cat/Cow Pose to practice breath work. Breathing is so important during labor because it can help with pain management during contractions and helps to facilitate birth by ensuring a good flow of oxygen into your body and to the baby. Cat/Cow Pose is made of simple movements to incorporate into your daily stretching routine. For Cow Pose, the position helps to open the upper back, which may get tight as the body grows forward with the expansion of your belly. The Cat position can help to strengthen abdominal muscles in a safe way. You will want to avoid huge backbends during pregnancy. Keep your Cow tilts more subtle, and focus on the upper back versus the lower back. Look online for yoga videos led by reputable instructors specializing in prenatal yoga to follow proper form.

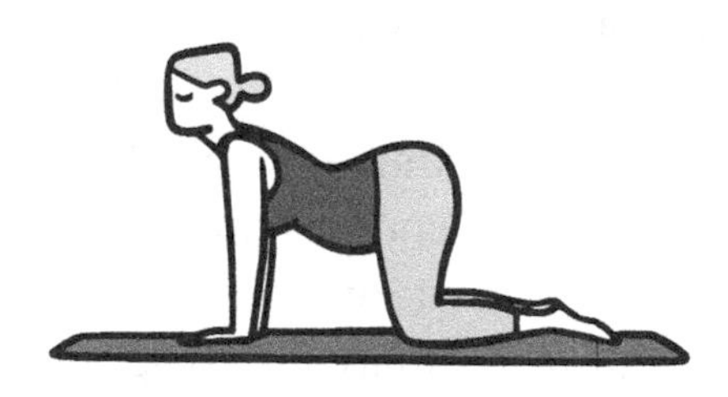

159 Do Side-Lying Savasana to rest and reinvigorate your body. Movement during pregnancy is important, but so is resting. Even at rest, your body is working incredibly hard to create life. Side-Lying Savasana is a pose that promotes rest and restoration. This pose is a great way to rest without being on your back (since doctors recommend not lying on your back starting at around twenty weeks). Lie on your left side and use props that you can hug and that will support your limbs. Let your body sink into relaxation as you breathe deeply.

••♦••

160 Try side plank variations to build core and upper-body strength. Side planks can help strengthen your core in a safe way, while also strengthening your arms—and you'll need that strength to carry around your baby. Balance is challenged during pregnancy, which is why it's important to modify some moves. Drop a knee in your plank to help provide extra support.

161 Begin your day with Child's Pose to gently stretch your hips, thighs, and ankles. Since sleep can be restless during pregnancy, starting your day with movement can help wake up your body and get it into alignment for the rest of the day. Try Child's Pose once you get out of bed. Kneel on the floor with your toes touching and your knees spread wide apart. Exhale and slowly lower your torso between your knees. If there isn't enough room for your belly, move your knees wider until there is space. If comfortable, rest your forehead on the floor. You can also extend and reach your arms forward, resting your hands on the floor forward of your face, or rest your arms at your sides with your palms facing up. This pose can help stretch your hips, thighs, and ankles, and can also provide calm to help relieve stress and fatigue as you start your day.

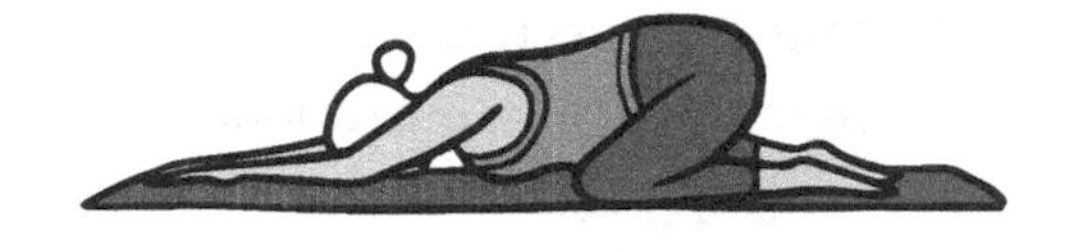

162 Try Happy Baby Pose early in your pregnancy to stretch your inner groin and back spine. We can't guarantee that doing Happy Baby Pose will lead to a happy baby, but it can lead to a happier mama, and that's the first step to a happy baby. This pose can gently stretch the inner groin and back spine, but it involves lying on your back, so only do it when your doctor says that it is okay. Lie on your back with a neutral spine and bring your knees gently toward your chest. Reach your arms through the inside of your knees and gently hold the outside edge of each foot with each hand. Press your tailbone down into the floor and pull down slightly with your arms.

••✦••

163 Don't stretch yourself too far. Pregnant women have an increase in relaxin, a hormone that relaxes joints and ligaments in the body. This is helpful for childbirth but can cause muscle strains and pulls during pregnancy. While doing Pilates or yoga, don't stretch beyond your pre-pregnancy abilities, as this may cause injury. Also, be aware that relaxin can remain in your body well after childbirth, so don't rush back into strenuous stretching.

Tips for Battling Morning Sickness

One of the most common discomforts of pregnant women is morning sickness. If you suffer from morning sickness, you may discover that it actually can strike at any point in the day, not just during the morning hours. While it's often associated with the first trimester, some women see it return in the third trimester, or battle it for all nine months. If you are experiencing extreme nausea and are having trouble keeping food or water down, speak with your doctor. For standard morning sickness, these simple tips may help.

164 **Make electrolyte cubes.** Can't even keep water down? Freeze electrolyte drinks (like Powerade, Gatorade, or coconut water) in ice-cube trays or in ice pop trays, and suck on these to stay hydrated.

165 **Pick one or two things you can stomach and repeat them.** Don't feel bad if that thing is a bagel or a bag of chips: This will pass, and eventually you'll consider eating a vegetable again.

166 **Keep snacks on your nightstand.** You have permission to snack in bed! Store crackers or pretzels next to your bed and eat them as you get into bed each night and before you get out of bed in the morning. If you wake up feeling nauseous at 3 a.m., see if you can eat one or two then too.

167 **Eat off smaller plates and bowls to encourage you to eat smaller meals.** Graze throughout the day with smaller meals instead of a big breakfast, lunch, and dinner. Eating from smaller plates and dishes can result in eating a smaller quantity at each meal.

168 **Eat ginger.** Ginger is a root known for its ability to soothe stomachs. Go for whatever form you prefer, including ginger chews, ginger tea, or even ginger supplements if you don't like the taste of ginger.

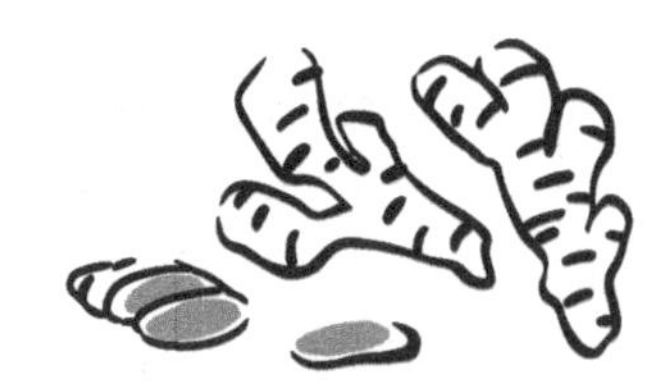

169 **Set out a day's worth of snacks and label them for specific times that you will eat them.** Eating snacks in between meals may keep nausea at bay because it keeps your blood sugar stable. When your blood sugar is too low and/or you have hunger pangs, or even if you overeat, nausea can worsen. That is why it is important to have frequent small meals throughout the day. Don't go more than two to three hours without eating something. If you tend to forget to snack, at the beginning of the day set out a bunch of snacks with labels for the time at which you'll eat them.

170 **Reduce your consumption of nausea-inducing food groups.** Cut back on fatty or greasy foods, sweet foods, spicy foods, and gas-producing foods, like cruciferous vegetables, beans, and dairy.

171 **Grab a bagel and increase your carb intake.** Bland, carb-focused foods might help you feel less nauseous. Eating fruits and vegetables is important to maintain a healthy diet, but it's okay to eat less if you're in the throes of morning sickness.

172 **Stop wearing perfume.** Certain strong smells may lead to nausea, so avoid them when possible. Now is a good time to stop wearing perfume and to make a friendly request that your partner or work neighbors do the same.

173 **Indulge in peppermint or lemon oil aromatherapy.** While some scents are going to make you queasy, others might bring you relief. Try peppermint or lemon oil, two scents that are said to relieve nausea. Some experts recommend holding off on the use of aromatherapy during the first trimester, so speak with your doctor before doing this.

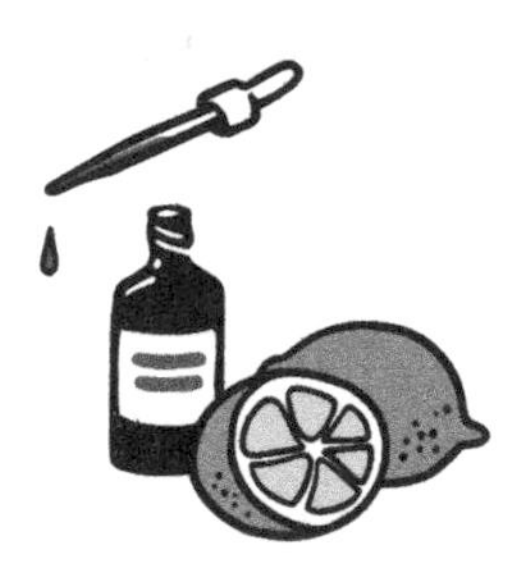

174 Swim for a low-impact workout. During pregnancy, your body may start to feel heavy, making your regular exercise routine more challenging than you're used to. If you're feeling weighed down, swimming is a great workout to explore during pregnancy. The water will support your extra weight and is a good way to stay cool while staying active.

175 Visit a float tank for ultimate relaxation and weightlessness. Float tanks are filled with warm water and hundreds of pounds of Epsom salt, which will allow you to effortlessly float and feel nearly weightless. It may help relieve back, spine, and foot strain; can aid in sleep; and promotes well-being. Speak with the float tank owner to ensure they know you are pregnant and request additional float devices, which may help you find a more comfortable position in the water.

176 Write down a list of skincare and haircare ingredients to avoid. Consult with your doctor if you are unsure of certain ingredients. As you do this research into what products and ingredients are okay and off-limits, keep an ongoing list in your Notes app so you can quickly reference it when purchasing new products.

••♦••

177 Shop for natural beauty and skincare products to avoid harmful ingredients. While you don't have to toss out your entire cosmetic bag, you should consider what you are putting on your skin during pregnancy. Review your current stash of moisturizers, perfumes, sunscreens, and acne treatments, as some products/ingredients may be off-limits during pregnancy and while breastfeeding. Where possible, switch to a natural or clean option. However, know that just because something is labeled "clean" or "natural" doesn't immediately indicate that it's pregnancy safe.

178 Keep a glass of water on your nightstand for middle-of-the-night wake-ups and to drink first thing in the morning. There are many recurring themes throughout pregnancy, and proper hydration is one of them. Each night while sleeping, you go for a long period of time without water. Hydrating with a glass of water upon waking can increase your alertness and provide an energy boost in the morning. Have a glass waiting on your nightstand so you can start sipping it as soon as you wake up. This is also helpful if you wake in the middle of the night feeling parched.

• • ♦ • •

179 Front-load your water intake, drinking most of your water in the first half of the day, to minimize middle-of-the-night wake-ups. With your bladder being compressed during pregnancy, it's no surprise that you'll find yourself needing to pee more frequently. To stay hydrated while also keeping the number of times you must get out of bed to pee to a minimum, aim to drink most of your daily water intake in the first half of the day. Slowly decrease the quantity you're consuming in the late afternoon and evening.

180 Take an Epsom salt bath to alleviate aches and pains. Mix about 2 cups of Epsom salt into a warm bath (remember to avoid very hot baths while pregnant). Epsom salt is said to soothe muscle aches and pains, reduce stress, and may aid digestion. Keep Epsom salt on hand for your postpartum days as well: Taking Epsom salt sitz baths can help to heal vaginal tears and hemorrhoids.

••♦••

181 Make a simple foot soak to reduce swelling. If you're not in the mood for a full bath or are nervous about hot water, instead focus on your feet. Draw up a soothing foot soak using warm water, about 1/2 cup of Epsom salt, and (if you want to make it extra fancy) a few drops of relaxing essential oils like lavender or rose. Best-case scenario, this soak will decrease foot swelling, and, if not, it's at least a relaxing ritual to partake in.

••♦••

182 Reduce foot swelling with a tonic water foot bath. If you don't have Epsom salt, try soaking your feet in room temperature tonic water. The quinine and bubbles may help reduce swelling.

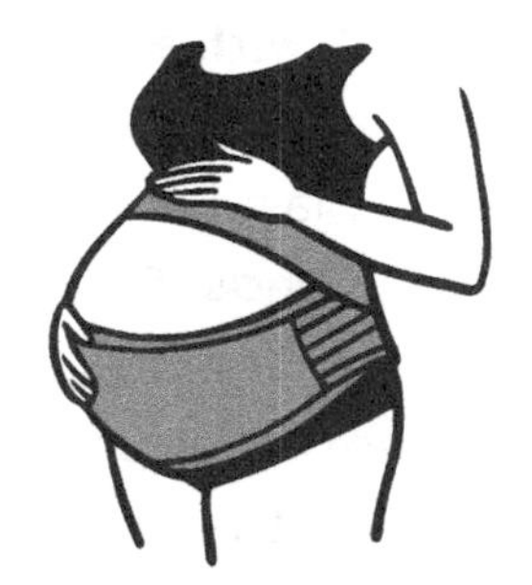

183 Get extra support with a pregnancy belt. Back pain is a common discomfort pregnant women experience, as is something called round ligament pain (that's a sharp pain around the lower belly or groin). To alleviate this pain, purchase a pregnancy belt or supportive belly band, which is a semi-structured garment that goes around your belly. It will provide extra support for the lower back and abdomen as your belly grows. Some women like to wear these all day, while others strap them on for workouts or long walks.

184 Bring a small pillow to work to provide lower back support. This pillow is not for napping on the job, though that does sound nice! Place it behind your back while sitting in your office chair to alleviate back pain.

185 Cool off at work with a mini desk fan. Feeling hot and sweaty during work? Since in an office setting you may not be able to blast the air-conditioning, take matters into your own hands. Prep your office space with a small USB- or battery-powered fan, your own personal cooling system. Post-pregnancy, these fans are great for clipping on the stroller on hot days as well (pointed at you or the baby!).

••◆••

186 Switch to a standing desk to alleviate back pain. Back pain may come and go throughout the next nine months. If you are at a job that requires sitting for many hours, request a standing desk, ideally one that can easily switch between a seated and standing height. This will allow you to switch positions throughout the day and will ensure you aren't sitting or standing for long periods of time.

••◆••

187 Make your own standing desk. If you can't get a standing desk, create your own with inexpensive furniture. Use a low side table on top of your normal desk for the monitor, and place your keyboard on a small shelf.

188 Curb constipation with a high-fiber diet. Constipation is never fun, but there are two times when it is extra uncomfortable: during pregnancy and after giving birth. To avoid this, eat a diet rich in fiber. Consume plenty of fresh fruits, vegetables, beans, bran cereals, and, of course, the classic standby, prunes.

••◆••

189 Stock up on stool softeners if you're experiencing bathroom struggles. If things are not moving along as naturally as you would have hoped, consider using a stool softener as a short-term fix. Check with your doctor to ensure you select one that is safe for your pregnancy. This is another item to keep on hand for the postpartum period—stool softeners will come in handy for your first post-labor bowel movement.

••◆••

190 Bring a stepstool into the bathroom to promote good pooping posture. Keep a low stool in your bathroom and place your feet on the stool when using the bathroom to help move things along naturally. By placing your feet on the stool, you will be sitting in more of a squat position, which can help ease constipation.

191 Use kinesiology tape to relieve common pregnancy aches. Kinesiology tape, often used by athletes to help alleviate pain, can be used as a creative way to minimize pregnancy symptoms and to relieve pressure and back pain. You can even use the tape to help relieve sciatica and reduce foot swelling. Look online or speak with a professional to ensure you are applying the tape correctly.

••✦••

192 Go to your routine dentist appointments to ensure good health. Pregnancy includes a lot of doctor's appointments. With so many visits to your ob-gyn, you may be tempted to halt all other health appointments, but don't skip out on your biannual dental appointments. During pregnancy, hormone changes can put pregnant women at an increased risk for gum disease, so it's important to stick with your regular appointments. Besides, you know what is even harder than getting to the dentist while pregnant? Getting to the dentist with a newborn. Make sure to tell your dentist that you are pregnant.

193 Reduce swelling by keeping your feet elevated on pillows, an ottoman, or a stepstool. Swollen feet and ankles are a common pregnancy symptom, but thankfully not typically a cause for concern (though if you are experiencing extreme swelling, discuss that with your doctor). When you are lying down, keeping your feet elevated can alleviate some swelling.

••◆••

194 Switch positions every forty-five minutes to lessen swelling. Another way to combat swelling is to consistently change your position. Try not to sit or stand for long periods at a time. Set a timer on your phone or have your smartwatch vibrate as a reminder to switch between sitting and standing throughout the day. Consider sitting for forty-five minutes, standing for fifteen minutes, and then repeating.

••◆••

195 Pack compression socks for travel to reduce swelling. Remember those compression socks mentioned in Chapter 2 as part of a maternity wardrobe? They are an essential travel accessory, as they will keep blood flowing and may reduce swelling while flying.

196 Plan your babymoon for the second trimester to take advantage of your energy boost. Getting away before the baby arrives is a great idea, but it's not as fun if you plan to go while experiencing extreme morning sickness or when you're feeling nervous about cutting it too close to your due date. The second trimester is typically when women feel their best and most energetic. Take advantage of this time and plan your babymoon sometime between weeks fourteen and twenty-eight.

197 Bring your own (empty) water bottle to stay hydrated while flying. Flying is known to make travelers dehydrated, so it's extra important that you continue to sip water throughout your flight as you travel during pregnancy. Bring your own water bottle (that you can fill in the airport after going through security) so you don't have to wait on the beverage service to get your first drink.

198 Splurge on a plane seat upgrade, if you can, for extra comfort. Cramped airplane seats are never fun, but this is never more apparent than during pregnancy. If your budget allows, treat yourself to an upgrade, even if it simply means a few extra inches to stretch out your legs.

199 Select an aisle seat for easy bathroom access and for more room to stretch. Because you will be doing a good job with your hydration, select an aisle seat while traveling during pregnancy. It will allow you to get to the bathroom without a hassle and will make it easier for you to stand up throughout the flight to stretch your legs.

200 Avoid super salty snacks while traveling to avoid bloating. It's important to have snacks available while traveling, but choose your snacks wisely. Consuming salty food while flying can make the bloating and swelling you might already have during pregnancy even more uncomfortable. Unsalted nuts, fresh fruit, dried fruit, and baby carrots are all good options.

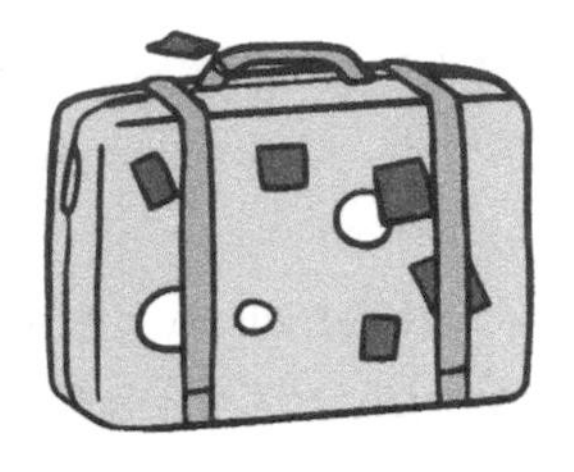

201 Ask for help with your luggage. Heavy lifting is not a great idea when pregnant, and though you may feel strong, hoisting a huge suitcase over your head is best avoided. Ask your partner, a flight attendant, or another passenger to help you. Even better, check your bag if possible.

••♦••

202 Treat yourself to a prenatal massage. You deserve some pampering, and a prenatal massage is a blissful way to lie back and relax. Find a reputable spa to ensure that you are in capable hands. Let the spa know that you are pregnant and request a pregnancy pillow or table. This will allow you to safely lie stomach-down during your treatment. Wait until the second and third trimesters, as many spas will not do them during the first trimester.

203 **Use a hot compress for easing round ligament pain.** Round ligament pain is described as a sharp or jabbing pain around the lower belly or groin, either on one or both sides. This is a normal part of pregnancy and usually occurs during the second trimester. While it is not typically a cause for concern, it can be very uncomfortable. Apply a warm compress to help alleviate the pain. Don't use extreme heat, as this can be dangerous to the fetus, and do not place the compress directly on your skin. Consider a microwavable heating pad, like a fabric one filled with rice. This way you can place the compress over the pain points, and the heat will gradually decrease over time. If you fall asleep, the compress will no longer be hot, making this a safer option than a plug-in heating pad or blanket.

204 **Roll to your side when getting out of bed to reduce diastasis recti.** Next time you get out of bed, avoid sitting straight up. Instead, gently roll your body to the side and then stand. This puts less pressure on your abdominal muscles and may reduce diastasis recti, the separating of ab muscles, which often occurs during pregnancy.

205 **Get acupuncture to alleviate some pregnancy symptoms.** Instead of getting poked with needles for all the various blood tests you have to undergo, look to needles to feel better. Acupuncture is an ancient healing method where tiny needles are inserted into specific parts of your body in a way that may potentially relieve you of certain pregnancy symptoms. Studies have shown acupuncture can alleviate morning sickness, lower back and pelvic pain, headaches, and sleep issues. Results of these studies are mixed, so it's not a sure thing, but acupuncture may be worth trying if you are struggling with these common pregnancy pains.

••◆••

206 **Slowly change positions to alleviate lightning crotch.** Ah, another unexpected less-than-pleasant pregnancy symptom you may experience. Lightning crotch is a sharp or shooting pain that you may feel in your vagina, rectum, or pelvis. The sudden pain is normal and may indicate that you are getting close to delivery (though it may occur at any time leading up to labor). Lightning crotch is caused by the pressure of the baby, and changing positions may help the pain to pass.

207 **Use a nontoxic deodorant or anti-chafe glide stick to prevent rubbing between your thighs.** As your body grows and swells, especially in warmer temperatures, you may experience an uncomfortable rubbing between your thighs when wearing dresses or skirts. You can use your nontoxic deodorant to help prevent chafing. If you'd prefer to keep your deodorant for your armpits, you can use an anti-chafe glide designed for runners.

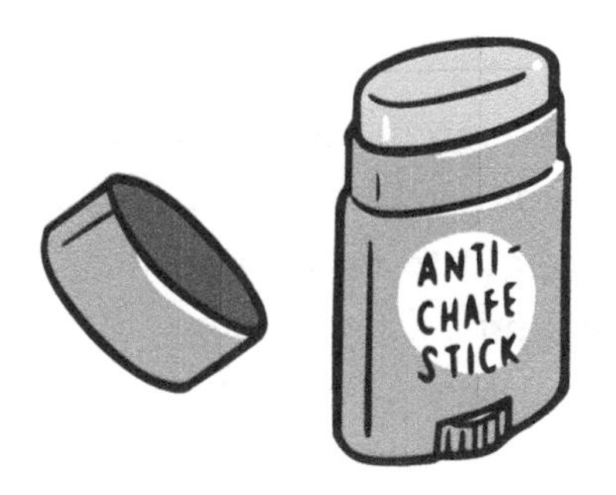

PARTNER HACKS

Make Your Pregnant Partner As Comfortable As Possible

208 **Offer her a nightly foot massage.** Encourage your partner to put her feet up at the end of a long day so you can rub them. Swollen and achy feet are common during pregnancy, and a nice foot massage can do wonders. Avoid pressing the inside and outside of both ankles, as that pressure may encourage uterine contractions.

209 **Look up pregnancy-safe stretches and help her with them.** With an ever-changing body and extra weight to carry around, your partner is likely feeling stiff and sore. Stretching can help. Look up stretches that are safe for pregnancy and help your partner get the most out of these moves. Keep in mind that women's bodies are more flexible during pregnancy due to an increase in relaxin, so be careful. Make sure she isn't stretching beyond her pre-pregnancy flexibility.

210 **Let your partner set the pace when you go for walks or runs together.** Staying active is helpful during pregnancy, and going for jogs or walks together is a great way you can support her. You may notice your partner's pace has significantly slowed down and continues to get slower the further along in the pregnancy she is. Don't rush the pace—go as slow or as fast as your partner is comfortable with.

211 **Draw her a warm bath.** A soothing warm bath is just what your pregnant partner might need. This can help ease muscle aches and is also an opportunity for her to relax. You'll want the water temperature to be close to body temperature, so aim for 98.6°F or cooler. If you're adding bubbles or essential oils, make sure they are safe for pregnancy.

212 **Do the heavy lifting.** Your partner may feel like she can lift and lug just like she did before pregnancy, but that doesn't mean she should. Whenever you can, take over the heavy lifting around the house and when you're out doing errands.

213 **Take over all the household cleaning.** Not only is it uncomfortable for your pregnant partner to be kneeling down to scrub a bathtub, but the chemical exposure can be dangerous too. This is the time to not just do your fair share of the chores; it's also the time for you to do all the cleaning.

214 **Take out the trash to keep your house smelling good.** Take out the trash in all rooms of your home and do it more often than you typically do. Your pregnant partner may be more sensitive to smells, and a full trash can might set off her nausea.

CHAPTER 4

Staying Strong Mentally

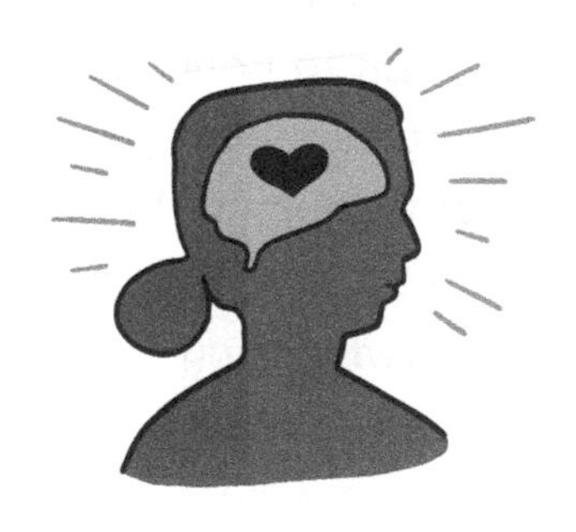

For some women, the emotional roller coaster of pregnancy may be just as exhilarating as the physical ride. Emotionally, you are going through a lot, with the changes to your body and lifestyle, hormonal changes, as well as mentally preparing for what's ahead when these fortyish weeks are over. Your whole life is about to change (in an amazing way!), and every day of your pregnancy is getting you one step closer to welcoming your newest family member.

Don't rush past your emotions during pregnancy. It's important to honor the way you are feeling, and also to do what you can to enjoy these precious moments. In this chapter, you'll learn the hacks that will help you find peace during this overwhelming time, including breathing exercises, practices to reduce stress, and other actions and check-ins you can do that will allow you to enjoy your pregnancy and look back on it with fondness.

215 Take time with yourself to process and write down your feelings. Sit with your thoughts and give yourself time to really think about how it feels to be pregnant. There are a wide range of normal responses to pregnancy, from happy and excited to scared, nervous, sad, stressed, and beyond. Whatever you are feeling is okay to feel. Don't rush past these feelings. Acknowledge your emotions and understand that they are valid.

• • ◆ • •

216 Download a meditation app to practice regularly. Meditation is a way to train your brain to clear your thoughts, which can lower stress and anxiety. Adding meditation practices to your daily routine can help you connect with your body and mind during pregnancy. Some research even shows that meditation helps women to prepare for labor and may result in a lowered risk of postpartum depression. Low-cost meditation apps you can use from home can help you jump-start your practice in as little as a few minutes each day. Use general meditation guides or sign up for pregnancy-specific meditation programs.

217 Write down a list of things you can control in life and focus on these things. You do not have a lot of control over some aspects of your pregnancy and childbirth, like when you'll go into labor and what your labor will be like. But there are things in life you *can* control. Focus your energy on those things, and this may make you feel more in control and at ease. Try not to stress over the things that you have no power over.

• • ♦ • •

218 Discover your emotional triggers by tracking your moods. Are there certain things that make you anxious and other things that make you calm? Write all these things down and try to do more of the calm-inducing actions and activities. If something is causing you stress, think about why it's making you feel that way and how you can alter the situation or your reaction to it.

219 Make a to-do list to keep track of everything. Preparing for a baby's arrival is a lot of work. Make sure to write it all down so you remember things and can celebrate your progress. Create an ongoing to-do list or make multiple to-do lists categorized by month or trimester. If you are feeling mentally overwhelmed and are having trouble quieting your mind, the practice of writing down your to-do list may take some of the burden off your mind and will allow you to relax.

220 Prioritize and rank action items on your to-do list. Once you've made your to-do list, prioritize your list and rank each item in order of importance. This practice may make you realize that some items at the bottom of your list aren't essential and don't need to be done. If that's the case, don't waste your mental or physical energy on those items.

221 **Assign some of your action items to other people.** Some people prefer to tackle their entire list solo instead of taking the time to delegate items, but now is not the time to do it all on your own. They say it takes a village to raise a child, and that begins with pregnancy. If you have a supportive village that wants to help, this is a great time to let them lend a hand. Is your mother asking what she can do? Does your best friend want to find cute crib sheets? Put them to work. It's also great practice if you're not used to asking for help. Asking for help will also be important as you bring home your newborn.

222 **Tackle only one small item a day or week.** Your long list might be overwhelming, even after you delegate certain items. Break your list down into small action items and tackle one item a day, or even one item a week. Accomplishing a task and crossing it off your list will make you feel more in control and more productive.

223 **Cry it out.** No, not the baby—you! Your hormones are fluctuating, and you may experience intense mood swings. Perhaps you find yourself crying more than you used to. Don't hold your tears in; it can be a nice release to let them out. Always carry a travel pack of tissues, just in case.

••◆••

224 **Use essential oils in your bath or with a diffuser to promote a calm mind.** Check with your doctor to be sure it's safe, and then consider using essential oils. Lavender may alleviate stress and depression, ylang-ylang can lead to calmness, and neroli may reduce anxiety. You can use diluted essential oils dropped into a bath or with a diffuser. When using a diffuser, make sure you are in a room with proper ventilation and don't use it for more than fifteen minutes at a time. Some doctors suggest avoiding essential oils early in pregnancy, so this may be something you want to save until you are further along. And remember, not all essential oils are safe for pregnancy, so do your research and check with your doctor before use.

225 Schedule a friend date to nurture your friendships. Speak with a close friend or two about how you're managing pregnancy. At first it might feel scary to be vulnerable, but the more you speak about your feelings, the less alone you will feel. Setting a special date and time will ensure you have dedicated time for you both to share your emotions. Maybe your friend experienced similar feelings and can share their coping mechanisms, or vice versa. Even if not, you will feel less alone in whatever you are feeling, and your community will be able to better lend support.

• • ♦ • •

226 Set aside uninterrupted time each day or each week to talk to your partner. Don't let your emotions build up. Talk about how you're feeling, and discuss your fears, excitement, and everything in between. Vocalize your moods often. If you have a change in mood, make sure to tell your partner. By speaking about your emotions and moods often, those closest to you can monitor when changes occur and can offer support if needed. Don't wait until things feel unsustainable to speak up.

227 Educate yourself about the signs of depression. General mood swings are very normal during pregnancy and are not necessarily something you need to be concerned about. However, if you are experiencing symptoms of depression, you will want to consult with your doctor. Know the signs to look out for, which include but are not limited to trouble sleeping, changes in appetite, struggles to concentrate, loss of interest in things you previously enjoyed, feelings of guilt, and thoughts of hurting yourself or the baby.

228 Send your partner articles on recognizing the signs of depression. It can be hard to see the signs of depression in yourself, so it's important that those around you also know the signs. Educate your partner on the signs of depression, as they will be the first line of defense in seeing the signs in you and can help you to act when needed. This is important during pregnancy and postpartum.

Easy Ways to Avoid Pregnancy Brain

Are you struggling to find your keys, can't focus during your work brainstorm, and completely forgot about your doctor's appointment? Blame it on pregnancy brain. While some dismiss pregnancy brain as a myth, there is research to support that there are real changes in the brain during pregnancy that can lead to forgetfulness. While it's perhaps impossible to avoid these changes, here are some tactics that can help keep your memory and brain sharp during pregnancy.

229 **Forgo multitasking.** It may feel like you can get more done if you multitask, but it's more likely that you'll lose focus and, in the end, will get less done. Avoid doing more than one thing at a time, and instead put all your focus on one task. Give it your full attention, and once that task is done, move on to the next.

☑ 1. *Wash dishes*

☐ 2. *Laundry*

230 **Repeat things out loud to help with your memory.** The more you say things, the more likely you are to remember them. When meeting a new person, repeat their name back to them out loud. If you're walking into a room to grab something, say out loud what you're going to get.

231 **Grab a pen to write everything down before you forget.** With so much on your mind, don't expect to remember it all. Instead, write everything down. And we do mean everything, including things you've never forgotten before. Partner's birthday? Write it down. Grocery list? Write it down. There's a lot going on in your head, and the more you can put down on paper, the less pressure you'll put on yourself to remember it all.

232 **Use your phone's camera to remind yourself of certain things.** Take pictures whenever you think there might be a chance that you'll forget something, like where your car is parked or which gym locker your gear is stashed in.

233 **Give items a home so you lose less.** Scrambling to get out of the house but have no idea where your keys are? Now is the time to give all essential items, like your bag, your keys, and your phone, a set home. Make it a routine to put these items in the same place every time you enter your home, and you won't end up finding your keys in the freezer (hey, it happens). Leaving the house with a newborn is a future challenge you'll be facing, and getting into a good routine of leaving your items in the same place now will also help you down the line.

234 **Set alarms and notifications so you get to appointments on time.** Stick to your schedule and get to appointments on time with the help of your phone's alarms and notifications. And remember that things might take longer these days, as you're moving at a slower speed. Set alarms that give you ample time to prepare and arrive on time.

235 Recite pregnancy mantras to feel empowered. Mantras are words, phrases, or short sentences that you can repeat to yourself that make you feel empowered and in control. Make a list of pregnancy mantras that you connect with. Repeat these throughout the day. Some examples include "My body was made for this," "I am doing the best for my baby," "I won't be pregnant forever," "I am a strong woman," "I am beautiful," "My baby will come when they are ready." Choose what resonates best with you and repeat it several times throughout the day.

••◆••

236 Post your mantras around the house to remind yourself of them. Keep your mantras top of mind by strategically placing them around your house and other places where you will see them often. Place notes on your bathroom mirror, on your nightstand, and in your favorite work notebook. When you spot them, they can provide a mini confidence boost.

237 Make an appointment with a therapist. Whether you've gone to therapy in the past or this would be your first experience, now is a wonderful time to visit a therapist. By speaking to a licensed professional, you are making your mental health a continued priority during pregnancy and beyond. You don't need to wait until something is wrong—the experience of pregnancy itself means you have plenty to discuss.

••◆••

238 Write down a list of all the things you are doing well and use it to practice positive self-talk. The way you speak to yourself impacts how you feel. Consider your current inner dialogue. Are you praising yourself and admiring what a good job you're doing, or are you upset with yourself for minor slipups? If you were talking to a close friend, how would you respond if they told you about the slipups? Be sure to speak to yourself in the same positive way. If that positive self-talk is buried deep and is hard for you to easily access, take a moment and write down the things you are doing well and things you like about yourself. If you ever feel your inner dialogue wavering, refer to your list as a reminder of how amazing you are.

239 **Practice a simple grounding exercise to help stay present.** There is a lot to think about while pregnant. At times your mind may go into overdrive with everything that you need to do and everything that's about to happen in your life. If you feel your mind wandering far into the future, pulling you from present-day reality, bring yourself to the present moment with a simple grounding exercise. Put your feet on the floor and notice the ground around you. If possible, take your shoes off and place your bare feet on the ground. Notice the way the ground feels and visualize roots growing from your feet into the ground.

• • ✦ • •

240 **Try the 5-4-3-2-1 technique to tune in to your senses.** This easy mindfulness idea can help you tune in to your senses, calm your thoughts, and bring you into the present moment. First, notice five things you see, then four things you can feel, then three things you can hear, two things you can smell, and one thing you can taste. Either do this in your mind or speak the things out loud. This list-making will take your mind off things stressing you out or making you uncomfortable and can bring you more into your present time and surroundings.

241 Introduce yourself to other expectant moms at yoga or in the doctor's office to build community. Even if you have plenty of friends with kids, they aren't going through pregnancy at the same time as you. It can be challenging for these women to look back on their past pregnancies and clearly remember the struggles and emotions. While these friends can be a great source of advice, also seek out friends (current or new friends) who are also pregnant. You can vent to each other and share tips. These moms-to-be will also act as your support system when you're a new mom. Find these women at your weekly prenatal yoga or Pilates class, strike up a friendly conversation with other pregnant women in your doctor's waiting room, exchange numbers with other couples at your child-birth class, or join local online groups that can connect you with nearby expectant moms.

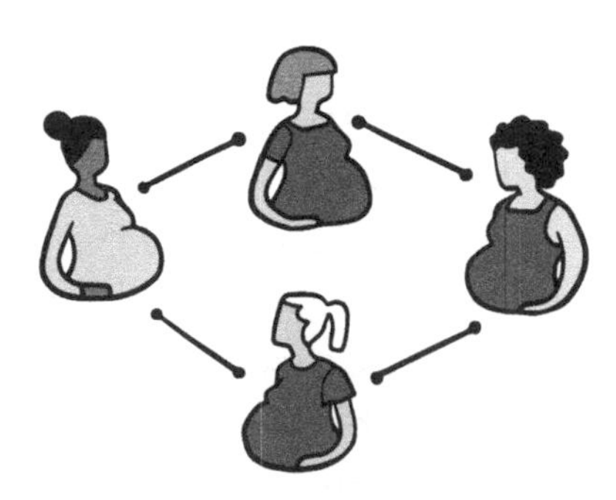

242 Experiment with 4-7-8 breathing to create a longer exhale. Shallow breathing isn't ideal, but that's what your body resorts to when you're stressed. A technique called 4-7-8 breathing can help you increase your exhale time, which allows your nervous system to slow down and can decrease anxiety. To do this, simply breathe in for four counts, hold the breath for seven counts, and exhale for eight counts.

••◆••

243 Leave your phone in another room at night so you don't get sucked into late-night Internet deep dives. Every ache and pain you're feeling can be scary, and it can be even scarier when you fall into a late-night Internet search session, attempting to self-diagnose on sites that may or may not be reputable. There are a lot of aches that you'll feel during pregnancy that are nothing to worry about—but if you are concerned about something, talk to your doctor instead of trying to search for an answer yourself.

244 Think about what you typically accomplish pre-pregnancy and then cut that in half to create realistic expectations for yourself. Pregnancy is a beautiful thing, but it is also incredibly demanding on your body and mind. Don't expect yourself to operate at the same capacity that you did pre-pregnancy—much of your energy and mindshare are rightly being directed toward the baby. Acknowledge that you are working hard and that you can only do so much. It is okay to slow down, to take a break, or to take a nap. Don't have high expectations of what you can accomplish right now.

••♦••

245 Keep an ongoing list of questions in your phone to address with your doctor. Questions are bound to pop up during your pregnancy. By the time you're at the doctor for your monthly or weekly visit, it can be hard to remember exactly what those questions were. If you forget to ask them, you'll likely be worrying about them for another whole month. Keep a list, either on paper or in your phone, that you can quickly add to and reference at each visit. You'll ease your mind having these questions answered regularly.

246 **Use prepared answers to say no to activities and reduce your responsibilities.** Trying to do too much and saying yes to every favor, activity, and outing that arises can take its toll on you mentally. Now is the time to scale back. Say no to things, even if it is the type of thing you would normally jump on board with. Think about whether you're saying yes to these things because you really want to do them or because you feel like it's something you *should* be doing. Focus on what you truly care about and skip the rest. So you're not caught off guard, have some prepared answers in mind for when things pop up. Some ideas: *Unfortunately, now isn't a good time for me. I would love to help, but perhaps [insert name] would be more helpful in this situation? I hate to miss the event, but tonight I need to rest at home.*

• • ♦ • •

247 **Tune in to a comedy to lighten your mood.** With your fluctuating emotions, watching certain emotional programs can be triggering. If you find yourself crying while watching a particularly sappy commercial, it might be time to switch to a comedy. If heavy dramas are affecting your mood, turn on a lighthearted show or movie and enjoy a much-needed laugh.

248 Let go of guilty feelings by thinking about the root of why you are feeling them. It's okay to be a little selfish, especially right now. Do what serves you and your family best. If feelings of guilt pop up, think through why you're feeling this way and seek ways to break the cycle. Let's say you feel guilty for skipping a friend's birthday party. Are you feeling this way because you think you are letting your friend down, or are you feeling pangs of guilt because it feels like letting go of part of your former self as you move into your new identity as a mother? By digging into these feelings, you can get a deeper understanding of why you feel guilty and can work to be gentle with yourself.

249 Read a book unrelated to pregnancy and parenthood for a little escape. It's amazing that you are reading this book, and yes, keep reading! It is also a great idea to add another genre to your daily or nightly reading routine. Pick a book that is unrelated to pregnancy and parenthood and is purely for pleasure. You're probably thinking about your pregnancy a lot, and reading for pleasure can be a nice escape, even if it is for just ten minutes a day.

250 Play relaxing music before bed to create a serene bedtime routine. It can be hard to function without proper sleep. You may find it is impossible to focus, you may become more forgetful, and you may lack the energy needed to get through the day. Getting into a good bedtime routine can help you both physically and mentally. Start your wind-down before you actually want to be asleep and find a routine that helps you move into sleep mode. A few elements that might help your bedtime routine: Stop using electronics at least thirty minutes before bed, leave your phone in another room, dim the lights, play relaxing music, read a book, and sip on a warm, calming beverage.

• • ♦ • •

251 Test out your baby's sound machine to help get a quality night of sleep. White noise can help you fall asleep faster and stay asleep. Sound machines are excellent for babies, and hopefully you have one on your baby registry (for more registry tips, see Chapter 5). If it arrives before your baby does, give it a spin yourself. White noise can help block out distracting sounds and provides a soothing backdrop as you nod off. If white noise isn't for you, some machines offer nature sounds, like gentle rainfall or ocean waves crashing.

252 Start a gratitude journal to focus on the good. If you notice yourself complaining more than you used to, this is normal—after all, you're experiencing a range of physical and mental ups and downs. Take some time each day to focus on those ups. Start a gratitude journal and write down one or two things you are grateful for each day. Entries do not need to be long or involved—they can be as simple as being thankful for the day's sunshine, your baby's health, or the call you received from a friend. Get your partner in on this activity as a new way to bond. This journal can help elevate your mood and increase your happiness as you focus on the good, and will also be a fun thing to look back on in the future.

••✦••

253 Keep a notepad and pen next to your bed to jot down middle-of-the-night worries. Is your to-do list keeping you up at night? Are you waking up in the middle of the night with new worries or concerns? Write down your thoughts because the act of putting them on paper may allow you to relax and get back to sleep. Use a physical notepad instead of the Notes app on your phone to avoid the screen light making you even more awake.

254 **Tune in to your own pregnancy, not the experience of other women.** Every woman experiences a unique pregnancy, and there is nothing to be gained by comparing yourself to others. Some bellies are big and round, some are tiny and barely there. Neither is better or worse; they are simply different. And while you may be battling morning sickness, your pregnant friend may be feeling like her best self. Don't dwell on her situation versus yours. Enjoy your own pregnancy and own your experience—don't get wrapped up in comparing your situation to others.

• • ♦ • •

255 **Set a social media time limit on your phone to help you disconnect.** Spending a lot of time scrolling? While it can be helpful to use social media to connect with other expecting moms and to get advice and ideas, you don't want it to lead to extra worrying or comparisons. Cut back on your social media consumption if it's making you feel anxious or stressed. iPhones allow you to set time restrictions on apps with just a few taps (Settings>Screen Time>App Limits>Add Limit).

256 Delete social media apps altogether if you're struggling to disconnect. If you're still scrolling too much and not feeling good as a result, delete the social media apps off your phone. It will take a lot more work to access the content, and eventually you may realize that you feel better without it.

••◆••

257 Go on a babymoon to de-stress. Vacations make everything better, right? A babymoon is the perfect way to get away from your everyday stresses and put your worries aside for a long weekend. It's also a wonderful time to connect with your partner, as it might be one of the last vacations that just the two of you take for a long time. Your getaway can be as simple as a one-night staycation at a local hotel, or as exotic as a bucket list trip you've always wanted to go on. Whatever destination you land on, let your doctor know your plans; then call ahead and let the hotel know you're celebrating a babymoon. They may welcome you with a special sparkling cider or keepsake onesie.

258 Create a work transition plan at the beginning of your third trimester. Your work situation may be weighing heavily on you, causing you extra stress whenever you think about everything that needs to be wrapped up at the office before you head off on maternity leave. Start your transition plan earlier than you think is necessary. You can update the plan as you get further along in your pregnancy, but starting early will ensure that it doesn't become a huge project you're rushing to finish toward the end of your third trimester, when your mind will likely be elsewhere. Plus, if you go into labor early, things will already be lined up. Make sure your coworkers know what your plan is and where to find the document so you can avoid juggling texts or emails from them with your newborn baby.

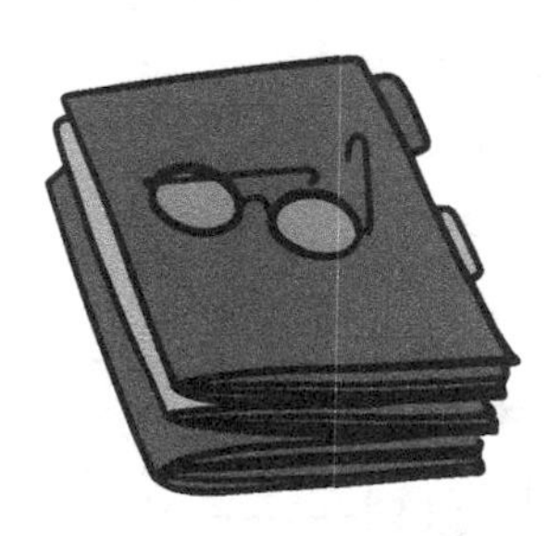

PARTNER HACKS

Support Your Partner Emotionally

259 **Tell her she's doing an amazing job and that she's beautiful.** Pregnancy is a beautiful thing, but your partner may not always feel beautiful. Make sure to keep the (genuine!) compliments rolling to keep her spirits and confidence high.

260 **Leave her love notes.** Put those sweet compliments down on paper, and leave them in spots that will surprise your partner and put a smile on her face. These don't need to be poetic pieces of work. Even a simple message like "You're beautiful," "You're going to be the best mom," or "Our family is so lucky to have you" can have a huge positive impact.

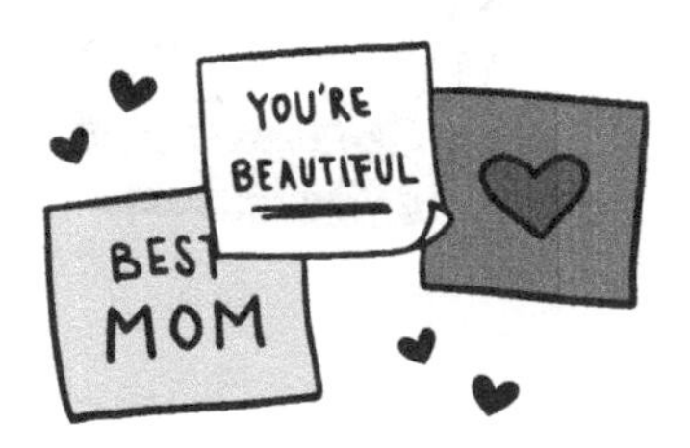

261 **Take a quiz online to learn your and your partner's Love Language.** Proper communication is important in any relationship, especially when you are preparing to bring a baby into the world. The Five Love Languages, developed by author Gary Chapman and outlined in a book by the same name, explain the different ways that people prefer to receive and show love. A quick online quiz can shed light on how you and your partner experience love. Knowing this about yourself and each other can strengthen your communication and overall relationship.

262 **Put your phone away when she's speaking to you.** Your partner is going through a lot emotionally, so let her lean on you (physically and emotionally), and listen to what she has to say. Quiet distractions around you so you can better focus and so she knows you are paying attention. As she vents, don't get wrapped up in a solution. Simply give her the space to speak through her concerns and worries. If she is truly looking for a solution, then you can talk about what those solutions could be, but if she is just looking for a place to vent and share, offer her that space.

263 **When she shares an emotion, share your feelings in return.** Share your own feelings as well—don't keep things bottled up. Yes, it's your partner who is pregnant, but you're going through this together. It's common for both partners to feel a wide range of emotions as they wait for their family to expand. Sharing your feelings will make you feel better and will also be a way to encourage your partner to speak more openly. You're probably experiencing some overlapping emotions, and this is a nice way to discover those and talk through them.

264 **Plan at-home activities, like a movie night, or low-key outings out of the house to keep her distracted.** Your partner likely has a lot on her mind and can also become particularly antsy in the final few weeks waiting for the baby's arrival. Keep her distracted from feelings of restlessness and worry by planning at-home activities, fun outings, or other low-stress distractions that will help keep her mind off aches, pains, and nervousness.

265 **Give her a hug and show affection.** Your pregnant partner may not feel like her most beautiful and glowing self during the various stages of pregnancy. You can help. Show her love and affection with something as simple as a hug and a kiss. Lift her spirits by telling her how strong she is and how much you appreciate her.

266 **Ask her what she needs.** Oh so simple, but when was the last time you asked your partner what she needs from you? Put this book down for a second and ask her now; then do what you can to make her life a little easier.

267 **Read about what perinatal and postpartum mood disorders look like.** Women can experience mood disorders, both during pregnancy and after. While many women experience mild baby blues, some situations are more serious. Educate yourself on the symptoms of these disorders. You will be the first line of defense for noticing when these disorders might arise and should be ready to assist your partner in getting proper help.

CHAPTER 5

Creating the Best Registry and Entering Nesting Mode

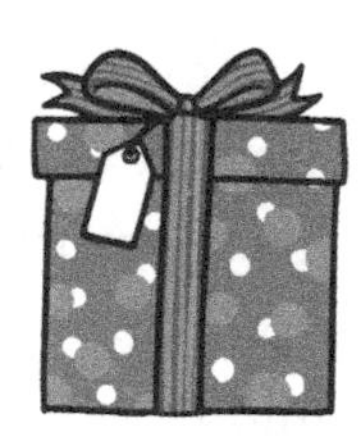

The amount of products out there for babies is mind-boggling. Do you really need *all* of those items? And how will you afford all of them? If you're lucky, you have friends and loved ones who will be eager to celebrate the baby with a gift—if so, setting up a registry is a handy way to show others your preferences. If you're mostly financing things yourself, you probably want to know what you'll really need. How many bottles, burp cloths, and onesies does a baby use, anyway? This chapter will guide you in creating the perfect registry, with hacks to gather all your gear, whether you're having three baby showers or none.

As you're researching baby gear and moving toward your due date, one day you might wake up with an incredible urge to clean and organize your entire house. Welcome to the nesting instinct! This is a very real phase that's meant to help you prepare your space for the baby. If you're feeling overwhelmed by all the potential work you could do, read this chapter to find hacks on the must-do nesting projects to tackle.

268 Take a deep breath and stay calm about your registry; don't get stressed by the process. Creating a registry can feel like an overwhelming task, but don't get too worked up about it. If you get a product you don't end up wanting, you can return it or give it to a mom friend. If you forget to add an essential item, you can always buy it for yourself or add it to your registry at a later point. It's great to have a well-thought-out registry, but it's okay if it isn't perfect. You will gather the necessary items you need for your baby, whether you end up getting something as a gift at your shower or pressing purchase on an online order as you head to the hospital.

269 Sign up for a universal registry instead of registering with multiple stores. If you're struggling to decide which store or site you should register with, consider using a universal registry. This means you don't need to stick to one retailer; you can instead select items from multiple retailers, and all the items will be housed within one big registry. You'll be able to add items to your registry from local shops, from *Etsy*, and from big retailers as well. Friends and family can easily access all items from one site. Search online to find a universal registry site that works for you.

270 Sign up for a registry that offers freebies.

Some registries offer a welcome kit of free products. It's usually made up of sample products and is a great way to discover brands and items you may not have known about otherwise. (If you don't end up using certain items, pass them along to a fellow new mom.)

• • ♦ • •

271 Choose items that fit your own lifestyle.

When you are getting recommendations from friends, reading blogs, or checking out ads, every item mentioned can seem important to own. The best way to choose is to think about your life and what you're most likely to use. Remember that every family is different. While one product may have been a lifesaver for your best friend, it might not be necessary for your lifestyle, your space, or your family. Your friend who runs marathons might love her jogging stroller, but you might instead prefer a backpack carrier that'll be great for the hikes you and your partner do regularly. Focus on items that will serve your family best.

272 Use the registry completion discount strategically. If you've got a few essential items left on your registry right before your baby is due, consider purchasing them with the registry completion discount. (Some registries will offer a completion discount, a special discount that you—the owner of the registry—can use to purchase items that no one bought for you.) For some registries, this is a one-time discount, so use it wisely with a strategic (and big) purchase.

273 Ask your mom friends for product advice. For first-time moms in particular, creating a registry can be overwhelming because of the amount of choices out there. Your mom friends are a great source of tips, product recommendations, and knowing which items are must-haves—that information can help you narrow down your choices. Every mom has their own opinion of what product is the best, so focus on asking friends that lead a similar lifestyle to you. They will be able to provide recommendations that will fit best with how you live your life and the budget you're working with. Create a document to keep track of all their suggestions.

274 Rank which registry items are the most important products to you. If your registry allows you to add special notes to items that are your "must-haves," be sure to do that. As much as you may want hair bows in every color of the rainbow, things like a car seat, a baby first aid kit, and a crib are actually essential items. By noting your must-haves, your friends and family will see the items you need most, which will help inform their purchases.

••◆••

275 Choose a registry with a flexible return policy. When registering for items, check your registry or each retailer's return policy. Even if you research products beforehand, it's likely that you will register for at least a few items that you won't end up using. The more flexible the return policy, the better. This allows you to deal with the returns when you have the time and energy to do so. (Worrying about and dealing with returns will be the last thing on your mind with a newborn.) Some companies allow for items purchased from your registry to be returned for up to 365 days.

276 Register for multiple brands/versions of the same item. Narrowing down which brand or style of swaddle, bottle, and pacifier to get can feel impossible. And really, since every baby is different with unique preferences, it *is* impossible to know what your baby will like before you try something. If you want to get five bottles, don't register for five of the same exact bottle. Instead, register for five different bottles. This way, you'll have options if your baby doesn't like some of the bottles. Once you know what they like, you can buy more (and if you haven't tried all five of the bottles, you can return unused ones).

• • ♦ • •

277 Include items on your registry that fall into a range of price points. Friends, family, and coworkers are likely working with varying budgets as they shop your registry. Provide items that cover a wide range of prices. Some registries even allow for multiple people to chip in toward the purchase of a larger gift (so one person doesn't have to pay, then collect money from the others). If you offer a wide range of price options, people will be more likely to stick to the registry when shopping for you.

278 Buy or register for one box of diapers. You will absolutely need a lot of diapers for your newborn baby—but don't go overboard buying them ahead of time. Babies have varying body types and sizes, and some diaper brands work better for some babies than others—but you won't know which brand you like best until the baby arrives. Start with one box of diapers and be sure that brand is working before buying in bulk.

279 Select items with zippers and magnetic closures, not buttons and snaps, to save time and frustration. Some baby clothing is incredibly cute but also poorly designed. Think about changing a crying baby's diaper in the middle of the night. Which seems easier to navigate, thirty buttons or one zipper on their pajamas? Keep this in mind when selecting clothing and opt for more zippers or magnetic items than buttons and snaps.

280 **Include items on your registry that your baby will use when they are a little bit older.** Newborn gear is extremely important, but eventually your baby will be out of the newborn stage, and it's nice to have some gear ready for those next stages. Consider adding things such as a high chair, sippy cups, and feeding utensils.

••◆••

281 **Register for only a handful of newborn clothes.** As adorable as newborn onesies are, they have an incredibly short life span. Within a few weeks, it's likely that newborn clothing will no longer fit (or will be stained with poop and spit-up)—and that's if it even fits your baby at all! (Some larger babies might jump right to a bigger size.) Select a few newborn items you love, but don't go crazy using up precious space on your registry for a ton of these items. Plus, people who purchase gifts off-registry often can't help buying tiny clothes...so you'll likely get more than you register for!

282 Register for non-material gifts, like dog walking, babysitting, and housecleaning. There are a lot of essential baby products to register for, but you can also get a little creative and add services to your registry. Instead of all material items, think about the various ways people can help you during the newborn stage. Consider adding things like dog walking, a home-cooked meal, babysitting, or housecleaning. These are things your friends can do for you (for example, nearby friends can bring you a home-cooked meal), or they can set these services up through a company (for tasks like housecleaning).

• • ♦ • •

283 Include travel items on your registry. Traveling with your baby requires a whole host of additional items, like a travel bag for your car seat, a travel stroller, and a travel crib. If you're planning trips during your baby's first year, consider adding these items to your registry.

284 **Add mom items to your registry.** It is called a baby registry, but it's okay to include products for mom as well. Think about what you need to help care for your baby and add those to your list. Look for nursing-friendly tank tops, pump parts, and childbirth recovery products.

• • ♦ • •

285 **Go to a store to test-drive certain items.** While you can select some items by viewing them online, other items are best seen and tried in person. If possible, find a baby store and stop by for an in-person review of certain products. Specifically, look at strollers and car seats. Check out how heavy and sturdy they are, and consider how easy or hard they are to set up and fold.

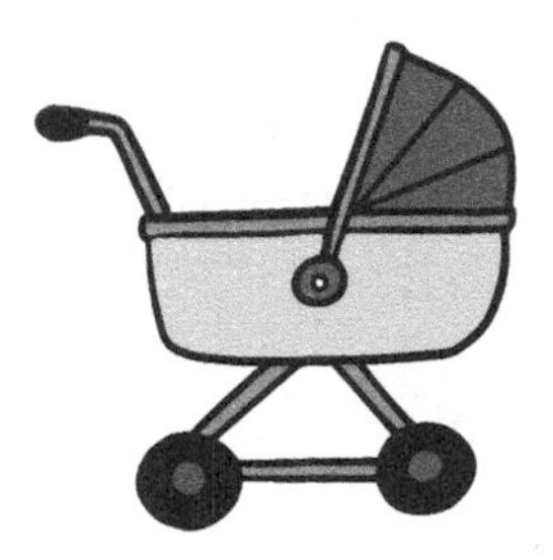

286 **Tell friends, coworkers, and neighbors that you're happy to get hand-me-downs.** Babies require a lot of gear, and the costs add up. If you are offered hand-me-downs you'll use, accept them. This will not only save you money, but it is also an environmentally conscious decision. Gather hand-me-downs early, and you can adjust your registry accordingly so as not to double up on certain items.

••◆••

287 **Set aside specific time to nest.** If you wake up one morning in the final weeks of pregnancy and have a huge desire to clean and organize your house, you are likely experiencing the nesting instinct! Make the most of that burst of energy and start to prepare your house for the baby. If you're having trouble finding time to nest, take a day off work or set aside a weekend to focus on it.

288 Write out a nesting to-do list. Instead of getting overwhelmed by tackling your entire house, go about it strategically. Decide which rooms need cleaning and organizing, make a list of tasks related to each room, and then prioritize them. Start with the most important rooms and items on your list. You could go into labor before your due date, so it's best to start with the most projects.

• • ♦ • •

289 Bring your breastfeeding-friendly and comfortable clothes to the front of your closet. Just as your wardrobe and most-worn items evolved during pregnancy, the same is true in the postpartum period. Your body is not going to magically return to its pre-pregnancy size (sorry!). Think about the items you wore in the second trimester. If they are seasonally appropriate for your first couple of months postpartum, make them easily accessible in your closet. Also consider moving comfortable loungewear and breastfeeding-friendly items to the front of your closet or drawers. If you switch around your closet with seasonal changes, think about doing this a little early so you're prepared ahead of time.

290 Hire help via online services for big projects. If it's something you can't do on your own, ask your partner for help, or hire someone to get it done. You can use online services to request help with a specific task, like building a crib.

••◆••

291 Start a low-stakes DIY project, like knitting a baby hat. Now is not the time to dive into any completely new projects or hobbies. Your energy levels might be low for big chunks of your third trimester, and you don't want any half-finished major work happening when you bring your baby home. If you're itching to do some DIY, take on a relatively easy project, like knitting a baby blanket or hat, or creating a piece of watercolor art for the nursery.

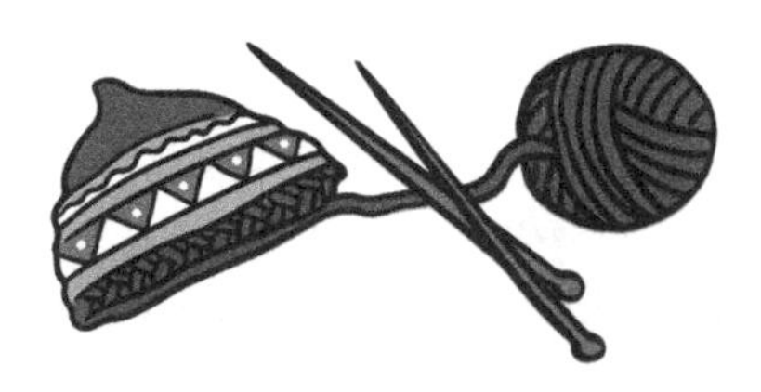

Your Nesting To-Do List

If the nesting instinct has struck, but you're not quite sure where to begin, here are some helpful tasks to get you started.

292 **Scrub down your refrigerator shelves and drawers.** When was the last time you gave your fridge shelving a good cleaning? Take everything out, wipe down all surfaces, and then put things back in an orderly manner. While you're at it, check the expiration date on condiments and other older items and discard as needed.

293 **Clean out your car.** Once you leave the hospital, you'll be headed to your car for the journey home with your new baby. It will be nice to get into a clean, junk-free car. Grab a garbage bag and dispose of any trash in your car and give it a quick vacuum.

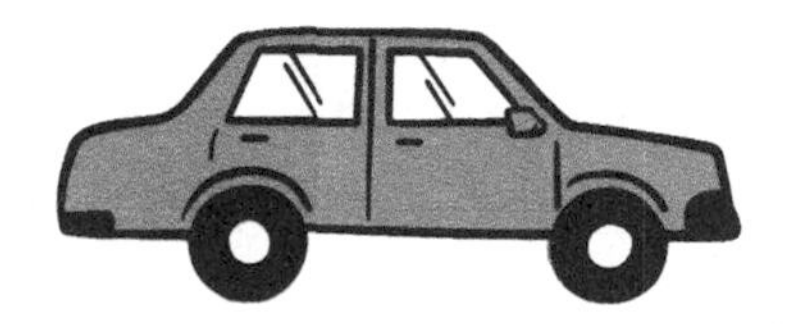

294 **Wash your duvet cover.** Give your duvet cover or comforter the washing it deserves, and while you're at it, make sure you have a clean spare set of sheets and towels on hand for the first few newborn weeks.

295 **Clear out your freezer.** Your freezer is a key area to clear out and organize. Fill it with freezer meals that will come in handy the first few weeks of parenthood when you will not have the time, energy, or desire to cook. If you plan to pump breastmilk and create a freezer stash, set up a designated area for it. You can use a small plastic box to help organize the milk.

296 **Refresh your bra and underwear drawer and toss uncomfortable items.** Go through your bra and underwear drawers and remove items that no longer suit you. Toss what you really don't care for or items that have seen better days. If you still like some items but they don't currently fit, they may fit again in the future, so place those in the back. Bring your looser, stretchy bras to the front, as these may work well for breastfeeding.

297 **Reorganize your nightstand and stock it with baby essentials.** Whatever essentials are currently in your nightstand may need to be temporarily displaced by baby items. These might include burp cloths, a pumping bra, baby wipes, diapers, pacifiers, and a spare swaddle blanket. See if you can make space for these additions.

298 **Organize your important papers in a tabbed folder.** A great low-impact nesting activity when you want to hang out on the couch is organizing important papers that you have in your home. Toss what you don't need, digitize what you can, and file everything else in an orderly way.

299 **Finish incomplete home projects.** If there are any half-finished projects in your house, now is the time to complete them. Saying "We'll just finish it after the baby arrives" is not a great approach. Maternity and paternity leaves aren't vacations, and taking care of your baby will be your number one priority, and will require a lot of energy. So go ahead and finish those projects now.

300 **Wash and organize some baby clothes and gear for sizes newborn to three months.** You'll want to wash and organize your baby's towels, bassinet sheets, and some clothing in sizes newborn up to three months. While you could wash all your baby's clothes, you may later realize that you don't need everything you have. If you wash a lot of newborn clothes, and your baby comes into the world already sporting size 0–3 months, you're stuck with all those unworn items. If you don't wash all of it and you keep tags attached, you may be able to return what you don't end up needing.

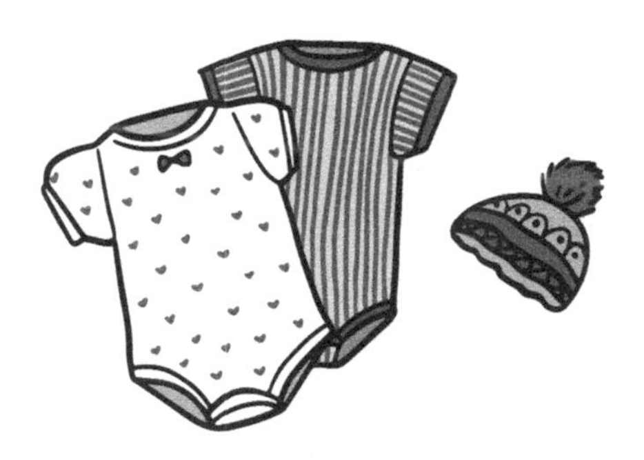

301 **Switch to a gentle laundry detergent.** You don't necessarily need to get baby-specific detergent, but it is a good idea to switch to a hypoallergenic laundry detergent designed for sensitive skin. Babies tend to have sensitive skin, some more sensitive than others. Consider making the switch and washing your clothes and sheets and all the baby gear in this detergent.

• • ♦ • •

302 **Set up two bins in the nursery for used baby clothes.** Babies grow really fast. One day their newborn onesie is huge on them, and the next day they've outgrown their nine-month wardrobe. Create a system now for staying organized later. One way is to have two bins in your baby's closet where you will place clothes as your baby outgrows them. One bin is for clothing you want to donate, and the other bin is for clothing you want to save. Once your baby outgrows an item, immediately decide if you want to save it (if you are planning for more kids), or if it will go in the donate bin. Once the bins are full, take the donate pile out for donation. Wash and store the clothes in the save pile, bagging them by size so they can await future use. If you have clothes that aren't in good enough shape to keep or donate, toss those in the trash.

303 Create a baby-feeding station in your living room. However you choose to feed your baby, designate a well-stocked space for this. Get a comfortable and supportive chair or glider and set up a table so that essentials will be within reach as you breastfeed, pump, or bottle-feed your baby. Essentials may include a feeding pillow, burp cloths, a water bottle, TV remotes, nipple cream, and a snack for you. Especially in the early days, babies will eat often and for long stretches at a time, so have your space prepared for this.

••♦••

304 Write a list of heavy-lifting tasks for your partner to do for you. As you nest, you may get carried away with everything you're accomplishing and may decide to take on some heavy lifting. Be very cautious, especially late in pregnancy. It can be dangerous to lift heavy items. This can lead to muscle pulls or hernias, or can even induce labor. Whenever you come across a task that includes lifting something heavy, write it down and give the list to your partner so they can safely handle those items.

305 Buy nightlights to illuminate your way around your house. During the first few weeks and months, it's common for babies to get their night and day mixed up, which means lots of nighttime care for you to manage. To help your baby adjust to night versus day, it's helpful to keep lights dim in the evenings. By strategically placing nightlights around your house, you'll be able to keep the main lights off while still safely moving around your house to feed and care for your baby.

306 Invest in a mini fridge for bedside milk storage. If you are planning to pump, you're going to need space to keep pumped milk. Middle-of-the-night pumping sessions are exhausting, and there is no need to make them more tiring with a trip to the kitchen fridge to store the milk at 3 a.m. With a bedside mini fridge, you'll be able to store milk with ease as soon as you're done pumping.

307 **Avoid stepstools and ladders.** As energized as you may feel to dust every corner of your house, keep yourself on safe ground. Avoid climbing ladders (or even short stepstools in your third trimester), as your balance is likely not at its peak.

••◆••

308 **Buy door latch covers for quiet door closing.** Consider every tiny sound in your home that might wake a sleeping baby. An often overlooked place is the sound made by opening and closing doors. Buy door latch covers—small pieces of fabric that loop over the door handles and cover the latch—for the rooms where your baby might be sleeping.

••◆••

309 **Make your own door latch cover with a thin piece of fabric.** To make your own door latch cover, you'll need a thin piece of fabric, elastic, and basic sewing supplies. Look up patterns and detailed instructions online.

310 Repurpose face masks as door latch covers. If you have fabric face masks that you previously used during a global pandemic, they work well to cover door latches. You may need to tighten the side straps on the mask to get a secure fit.

••◆••

311 Set a timer to limit the amount of time you spend on a task. As you should be doing throughout all of pregnancy, listen to your body and know when it's time to take a break. It's easy to get carried away with a task, but if you're getting tired, lie down and rest. Don't push yourself too hard during these intense weeks. To encourage rest periods, set a timer before starting a task. Once the timer goes off, take your break.

••◆••

312 Take stock of your pantry. Now is the time to toss expired or stale items, see what you're running low on, and restock. This will ensure that you're prepared for the newborn weeks when going to the grocery store will likely be low on your priority list.

313 Think beyond the nursery and figure out which rooms need work to prepare for life with a baby. You'll want to prepare your entire house for the baby, not just their nursery. In most cases, babies don't even sleep in their nursery for the first few weeks or months of life. Do you need to clear out a corner of your bedroom to fit a bassinet? Should you set up a temporary diaper-changing station in your room to make middle-of-the-night diaper changes as seamless as possible? Can you create space in the garage for the stroller? Should you make space in a kitchen cabinet for bottles?

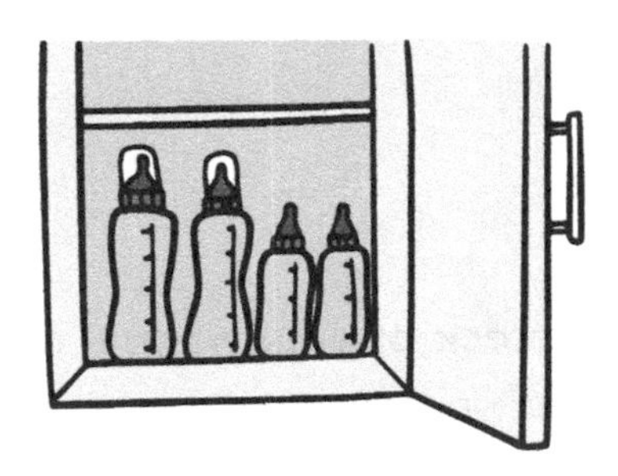

PARTNER HACKS

Join in the Nesting Fun

314 **Build the essential nursery furniture.** Your baby might not sleep in the nursery for their first few weeks or months of life, but it's still nice to have the bulk of the nursery set up and ready to go before they're born. Make sure the dresser is built early so you can organize and store clothes.

315 **Babyproof your biggest pieces of furniture.** It's not necessary to have your entire house babyproofed before your baby arrives, but there are some steps you can take now to avoid the work later (when you're caring for a baby). Make sure bookcases and dressers around the house are properly anchored to the wall.

316 **Paint the nursery so your pregnant partner can avoid the fumes and heights.** While most paint is safe for use during pregnancy, this is one of those tasks that you can do instead of getting your pregnant partner in a paint-fume-filled room and up on a ladder to paint.

317 **Have your partner give you a tour of the nursery.** If your pregnant partner is doing most of the nesting and organizing, you might need a little tour of the space to know where everything is. Take note of where pajamas are, extra diapers, wipe refills, and more. The better you know the space and the organizational systems in place, the more helpful you will be, especially during those first newborn weeks when your partner is recovering.

318 **Get an extra set of clean sheets ready.** Have a spare set of sheets and towels cleaned and ready to use once the baby arrives. It will be nice to come home from the hospital to a fresh set of sheets. You can either change the sheets before you head to the hospital (if your partner is spending some time laboring at home) or as soon as you return from the hospital.

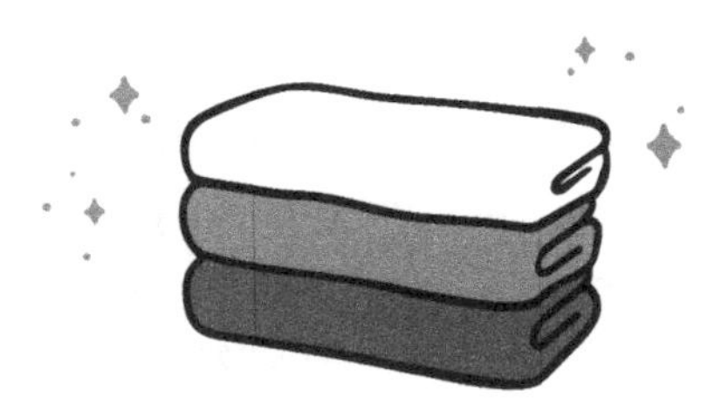

319 **Assemble the stroller and give it a test-drive.** If your stroller arrives in a box, take it out and build it before the baby arrives. Make sure you know how to fold and unfold it. Give your partner a demonstration as well.

320 **Keep your own to-do list for nesting action items.** Whether your partner is assigning you specific tasks, or you are brainstorming your own ways to prepare for the baby, write it down and keep adding to your list. When you have a free moment, see what items you can check off. Prioritize items that must get done before the baby arrives.

321 **Practice babywearing with a stuffed animal or doll.** If you plan to use baby carriers, give them a try before the baby arrives. Watch videos online to ensure you're putting it on correctly. You can use a doll or a stuffed animal to see how it will fit with a baby, and this will allow you to do practice checks to make sure the baby will be in the correct position with their airway open. This is a great partner task since a big belly will get in the way of your pregnant partner testing out the carriers.

322 **Practice inserting the car seat and have it professionally checked.** Install the infant car seat base in your car (or the convertible car seat, if you're using one). Hospitals will not allow you to leave without a car seat properly installed. A high percentage of people incorrectly install the car seat, so make sure you have it securely set by having a trained professional check it. Do this early in case your partner goes into labor before the due date. Some children's hospitals, police stations, and fire stations can perform a car seat safety check. Check what is available in your area and if an appointment is required. You will likely be responsible for putting the car seat in for the baby's first car ride since your partner will be healing from the birth. Make sure you know how to properly set it in the car by practicing a few times to boost your confidence.

323 **Minimize creaks and squeaks around your house.** Think about the unnecessary squeaky sounds in your house and how these may impact the sleep of a baby. Investigate all creaks and remove the ones that you can from doors, floorboards, stairs, and so on, using WD-40 or other appropriate methods.

CHAPTER 6

Preparing for the Big Day and Beyond

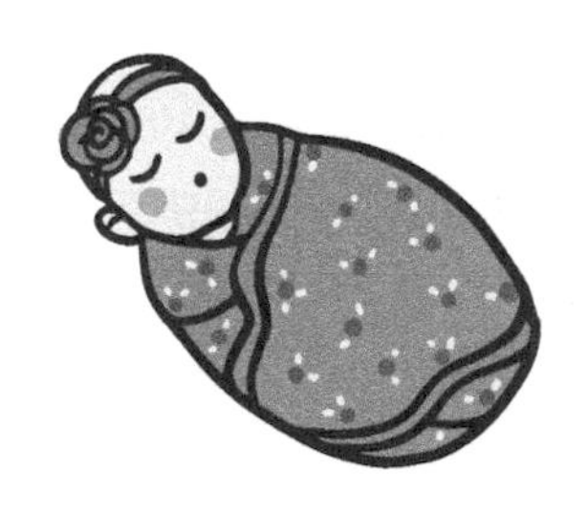

Welcome to the home stretch! Whether your pregnancy flew by or felt like it lasted ten years, you're nearly there. All that's left to do is prepare for labor, delivery, and bringing home your baby. Thankfully, this chapter is full of hacks to make this potentially overwhelming and stressful part of the process a bit simpler and more streamlined. Though it's truly impossible to fully prepare for what's ahead, you *can* do a lot to ready your mind, body, and home for the big day and beyond. You'll find ideas for how to get ready for labor, tips for putting the final touches on your home, suggestions on expertly packing your hospital bag, and more. You can do this!

324 Make a birth preference plan, write it down, and put it in your hospital bag. Take a few minutes to think through what you would like the birth to look like. Consider if you plan to receive pain medication, what type of atmosphere you'd like (dimmed lights, soft music, etc.), if you want to take a bath or take a warm shower, if you'll use a birthing ball, and so on. Write it all down and discuss it with your partner. Keep this list in your hospital bag so you and your partner can reference it when the big day arrives. You may also be able to send this to your provider in advance so they are aware of your wishes. (A note: It's good to have preferences, but it's very important to know that things might change and may not go the way you thought they would. Keep an open and flexible mind.)

• • ♦ • •

325 Keep your hospital essentials by the door during the third trimester. When the time does eventually come to head to the hospital, you may be in a bit of a daze. Don't forget all the essentials you want to bring with you. Keep your hospital bag and other important items by the door so you can quickly grab them on your way out.

326 Write down the rules of when you are supposed to go to the hospital, and keep the information handy. Each hospital has different guidelines for when you should arrive. Know your hospital's specific rules. Generally, it's something like if your contractions are coming around five minutes apart, each contraction lasts for one minute, and this has been happening for one hour, you can be admitted (5-1-1 rule). Know the rules for your hospital, and write them down for easy reference. When you do go into labor, it might be hard to remember with so many things running through your mind. If you think you are going into labor, call your hospital. If it's not your first baby, labor tends to move much faster, so you may need to head to the hospital on the earlier side. And remember, there are a lot of factors that go into when you should go to the hospital, like how far you live from the hospital, time of day, traffic, if this is your first birth, your baby's positioning, if you have gestational diabetes, and more, so make sure to call as soon as you think you are in labor so the hospital can tell you what to do.

327 Charge your tech items multiple times a day. In most cases, you won't know exactly when your baby will be born. Don't be caught off guard with dead batteries. Always do your best to keep your phone charged, and pre-charge other items that you plan to bring with you (like a speaker and good camera).

••◆••

328 Go on a hospital tour with your partner or labor support person. If your hospital offers tours, take advantage and go. Knowing where to park, the right place to check in, and having an idea of what the rooms look like will make for a smoother check-in and creates fewer unknowns when you head to the hospital for the big day.

••◆••

329 Call the hospital and see if you can request specific nurses. If this isn't your first birth and you've delivered at the same hospital for previous births, you may be able to request certain delivery and recovery nurses. Find out your hospital's policy and get your requests ready if you have them.

330 Sign up for an online childbirth class if in-person ones don't fit your schedule. Be as prepared as possible for labor and delivery. Having some sense of what might happen can give you peace of mind, and a childbirth class can help you be informed. There are a range of available classes, from quick one- or two-hour classes to online options to multi-week, in-depth offerings. Decide what is best for you so you can feel sufficiently prepared for the experience. For busy moms-to-be, sign up for an online childbirth class that you can take from the comfort of your own home.

331 Take an infant CPR course with key loved ones. It can be scary to think about choking and CPR with babies, but it's important to be prepared for these situations. Take an infant CPR class before the baby arrives—and have any caregivers join you. Have your partner join you, and if relatives and grandparents will be helping to take care of the baby, invite them along as well. While hopefully you won't have to put your learnings into practice, it's best to know the right steps to take in the event of an emergency. If you can't make it to an in-person class, there are budget-friendly online courses available.

332 **Take a basic childcare class.** Childbirth classes are helpful, but don't forget to learn about taking care of your baby! It's not possible to learn everything about taking care of a baby ahead of time, but don't worry; you will learn as you go. However, it is helpful to take a basic course to learn a few elements, such as how to swaddle a baby, how to soothe an upset baby, how to bathe a baby, general safety practices, and more.

333 **Gather contact information for night nurses, postpartum doulas, and sleep consultants.** Life with a newborn, especially your first baby, is a time when you need and deserve support. There are several ways to get this support, through things like postpartum doulas, sleep consultants, and more. You don't need to decide and hire these people before your baby is born. If you're on the fence about whether you'll need it, the best approach is to gather information before the baby arrives. Get recommendations from friends, reach out to conduct introduction interviews, and have your favorites noted. This way, if you do decide you want the help, you'll be ready to call on professionals without going through the research and interview steps with your newborn.

334 Hire a service to preserve your placenta and tell the hospital about it (if necessary). Some women choose to save their placenta and use it in a variety of ways. You can have it encapsulated, use it in smoothies, or bury it. If you want to use your placenta for something, make sure to hire the service ahead of the birth and make sure the hospital is aware of your plan.

••◆••

335 Practice your swaddling technique with a doll or stuffed animal. Snugly wrapping a blanket around your baby can help soothe them and can promote better sleep for the first few months of life. There are a few different swaddling techniques, and it can be helpful to practice these before the baby arrives. Look up videos online and work on your technique.

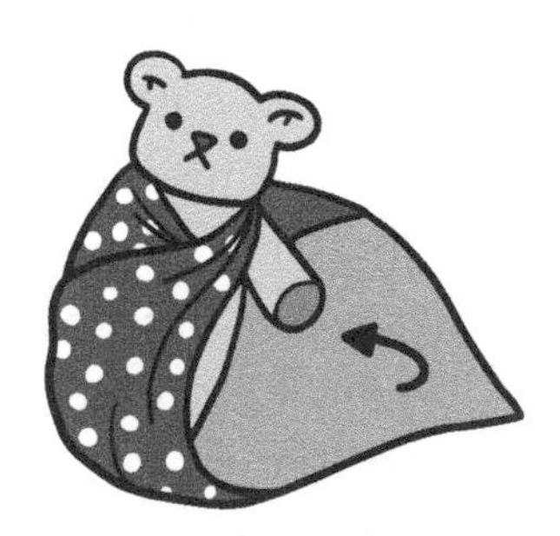

336 Schedule five-minute walks at several points throughout each day. You're in the home stretch of pregnancy, and those final weeks can be the toughest to find the motivation to exercise. Your body is big, you're probably tired, and you might be feeling weighed down. Do your best to keep moving, even if that means going for short walks around the block or even around the office. Mark these walking breaks in your calendar so you are reminded to get up and move around.

337 Consider having a "gentle C-section" if the option is available. If you are having a scheduled C-section, you may be able to request a "gentle C-section," which can include a transparent curtain so you can see the baby emerge and usually allows for skin-to-skin moments after the baby is born. The practice is meant to seem more like a vaginal birth instead of surgery. However, know that not all C-sections (whether scheduled or emergency) can allow for this, but it's worth researching and discussing with your doctor if it's of interest to you.

338 Do squats during commercial breaks while watching TV. Doing squats while pregnant can help your hips, glutes, and pelvic floor muscles to stay strong and active. And in labor, squats may help open your pelvis and aid in the baby's descent. The more you practice squats while pregnant, the more likely you'll have the strength and energy to do them during labor. An easy way to fit these into your day is to do them during each commercial break as you watch a show. If there aren't commercials, do them during the opening credits or during the beginning, middle, and end of a show.

••◆••

339 Gently bounce on a birthing ball while listening to a podcast or reading a book. A large inflatable exercise ball, or birthing ball as you may be currently calling it, is great to have for exercising while pregnant and also to prepare for labor. Sitting and bouncing on a birthing ball helps to strengthen core and back muscles and can help you maintain good posture. It may also relieve certain pregnancy aches and pains. Once in labor, using the ball can help open your hips and pelvis and minimize labor pains. Get in the routine of bouncing on a ball while at home, such as while listening to a podcast or as you read a book.

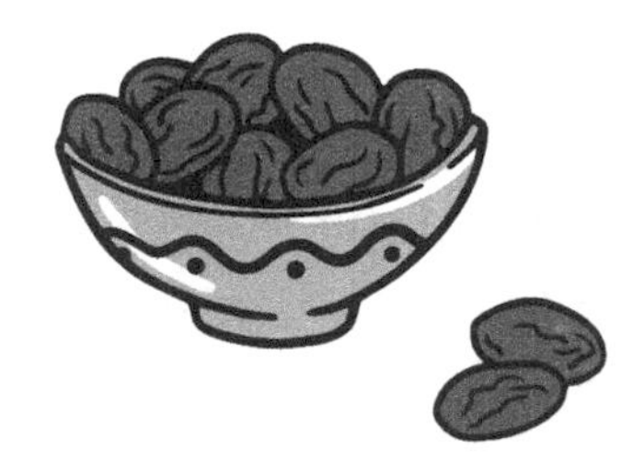

340 Eat dates daily to promote natural labor. If you have a sweet tooth but are trying to cut back on artificial or added sugar, dates are a delicious and healthy way to satiate your sugar cravings. Beyond that, some research supports the fact that eating dates in the third trimester may promote natural induction.

• • ♦ • •

341 Sip on red raspberry leaf tea to potentially decrease the amount of time you spend in labor. Some studies indicate that there are benefits to drinking red raspberry leaf tea, which is rich in vitamins and minerals. These studies suggest that it can strengthen the uterine walls and may even help your birth to proceed without artificial rupture of membranes or C-section. It also may shorten the time you are in labor. It is recommended to drink one to three cups a day in the third trimester.

342 Prepare freezer meals you can eat with one hand. Making meals ahead of time will save you a lot of hassle and money when you're home with a newborn. Think of what will be easy to eat with one hand (breakfast burritos are a great option). Once the baby arrives, you can simply toss your prepared frozen meal in the microwave and be eating homemade food within minutes. This comes in handy when you get sick of takeout.

••◆••

343 Make and freeze a batch of lactation cookies. If you plan on breastfeeding, lactation cookies are an excellent snack to have once you're home with your baby. There are certain ingredients that are said to boost milk production, like brewer's yeast and oats. Look online for lactation cookie recipes that include those ingredients, and then make and freeze some. Not only are they said to be good for milk supply, but they are also a very tasty treat you'll look forward to after labor.

344 Make a childbirth playlist and bookmark a backup playlist. If music is on your birth preferences list, make sure to have a playlist all organized and ready to go. Think if you will want upbeat, motivational tunes or low-key and calming sounds. Remember that labor can take a long time—and it may be unrealistic to make a twenty-five-hour playlist. If you pay for a streaming service, bookmark a few premade stations that you like so you can rely on those if your playlist ends and the baby still hasn't arrived.

345 Schedule a meet and greet with a pediatrician before your baby is born. Your baby will likely be making their first visit to the pediatrician within a week of being born. It will make life easier if you already have a pediatrician picked out and have already spoken to them to form a relationship. Also, if you have questions before that first appointment, you'll already have a point person that you can reach out to.

Items to Have in Your Hospital Bag

Around thirty-five or thirty-six weeks, it's time to get your hospital bag packed! Some items are an absolute must, while others are recommendations for a more comfortable stay. Have everything packed, and write down any last-minute items that need to be tossed in before you head out the door (like a toothbrush). Make sure to put that list on top of your bag as a reminder. There will be a lot on your mind as you head to the hospital, so don't rely on a clear head to remember those final items.

346 **An empty tote bag to fill with products from the hospital.** Pack an extra empty bag within your hospital bag, as you will be leaving the hospital with more than you arrive with (and we're not just talking about the baby!). While at the hospital, you can often stock up on newborn baby gear, including diapers, wipes, and receiving blankets. Plus, you can take home recovery products for you, like pads, disposable underwear, creams, medications, and lotions.

347 **A supportive pillow for comfortable rest.** You don't know how long you'll be at the hospital, and chances are, the pillows aren't quite as comfy and fluffy as the one you have at home. Pack your own to bring a little comfort to your hospital stay.

348 **Nourishing snacks, more than you think you'll need, just in case.** The hospital probably offers food, but if you have some favorites that you'd like to have for before and after the birth, pack them. Plus, some hospital cafeterias have limited hours, and if you're up laboring in the middle of the night, you're probably going to get hungry. Pack more than you think you will want; it's always better to have excess than not enough.

349 **Soothing lip balm to combat dry air.** Hospitals are notorious for having dry air. Dry, chapped lips can easily be soothed with a lip balm in your hospital bag.

350 **Hydrating clear drinks for an energizing boost.** Hydration is important during the strenuous experience of giving birth. The hospital will have water and other drinks available to you, but if there is a specific drink you will want, pack it in a cooler and bring it with you. Think about hydrating and fueling options. If you get an epidural, you won't be able to eat, but you can have clear liquids, so something energizing like coconut water is a good choice.

351 **Extra-long charging cords that will keep your devices charged and within arm's reach.** Keep your electronics well charged during your hospital stay with an extra-long charging cord. Your products will stay charging, and you'll be able to hold on to your phone while you're in bed.

352 **A battery-operated (or well-charged) speaker to keep the motivational tunes coming.** If you prepared a labor playlist, bring a speaker so you can listen to it with a good sound quality.

353 **A cozy robe, pajamas, and slippers for walking the hospital halls, and for first photos with the baby.** When you're sick of wearing the hospital gown and are ready to do short walks around the hospital halls, a comfortable robe and pajamas are the perfect thing to slip into. Dark-colored items work well, as you can expect a variety of stains from bodily fluid, both from the baby and from you during labor, delivery, and after.

354 **A comfortable going-home outfit for you and the baby.** You'll need both an outfit for you and one for the baby to head home in. For you, think loose, breathable, and comfortable. A ribbed tank maternity dress is a nice option, as this won't rub uncomfortably whether you have a vaginal or C-section delivery. For your baby, keep it simple with a one-piece newborn outfit.

355 **Hair ties and a headband to control your hair.** Labor can be a sweaty situation. Keep your hair somewhat tamed during the experience with a good headband and hair tie.

356 **Cooling face and body wipes when you need a quick and simple refresh.** Washing your face and showering after the birth of your baby will bring new life to your tired and overworked body. But you might not be up for that shower until a day or two postpartum. Plus, if you're experiencing a long labor, a refreshing wipe might be just the thing you need. Pack fragrance-free, organic face and body wipes for a quick refresh while in the hospital.

357 **A toothbrush and toothpaste for multiple days in the hospital.** You'll likely be at the hospital for at least twenty-four hours following the birth of your baby, if not longer. Your own toothbrush and favorite toothpaste are good to have around.

358 **Your birth preferences plan, as a reminder of what you'd like during birth.** Remember that birth preferences plan you wrote out? Add this to your hospital bag for easy reference by you, your partner, and your nurses.

359 Begin filling in your baby book while you're still pregnant. Were you given a sweet baby book as a gift? Don't wait until the baby arrives to open it up. Many baby books start with a section to write in before the baby arrives. Here you can enter guesses for the baby's birthdate and weight, share details about your pregnancy, and record your feelings and emotions as you wait for your baby's arrival. Get started on these sections before the big day comes.

• • ◆ • •

360 Ask someone to care for your other children ahead of time. If you have other children, figure out their care plan for when you go into labor. Decide who will watch them, pack their bag if necessary, and make plans for how and when the children will visit at the hospital to meet their new sibling. If the person doesn't usually care for the child, make sure to discuss any specifics of care. Make a backup care plan to be extra safe.

361 **Plan pet care.** Be sure you have someone ready to take care of your pets when you go into labor. Discuss any care specifics ahead of time (walk schedule, feeding times, etc.). And since the exact date you will go into labor is unknown, also have backup care planned in the event your go-to person is unavailable.

• • ♦ • •

362 **Write out a help/chore chart for guests visiting after the baby is born.** You might associate a chore chart with kids, but it's actually a great thing to have in your home for the first few weeks with the baby. If you have visitors coming over, they (hopefully!) will want to help the new parents. It can be awkward to ask for specific things, and if you don't feel comfortable asking, you can instead create a list and put it in a place where your guests will see it (like the refrigerator door). If a guest comes over and asks how they can help, instead of giving them a specific task, you can tell them to check the list and do whatever they'd like to do. Tasks like washing dishes, taking out the trash, walking the dog, and folding laundry are easy things for other people to do.

363 Sign up for auto delivery of baby essentials. There are a lot of things you will need frequently once the baby arrives, like diapers and wipes. Go ahead and sign up for auto delivery from an online retailer before the baby's arrival. This way, you'll already have your address and payment method set up when you want to order something. You can always change your delivery settings if the timing isn't right or if you want to swap out products.

364 Fill an online cart with remaining baby essentials and press Buy when the time comes. If you haven't yet bought a few baby essentials because you're waiting to see if they will be purchased off your registry, add the most essential items to an online shopping cart and select Save for later. Include things like diapers, wipes, a thermometer, burp cloths—the types of items that you will absolutely need when you return home from the hospital. Once you know the baby is on the way, you can simply place your order.

365 Prepare your birth announcement email list and start a draft message. If you plan to send an announcement to friends and family once the baby arrives, prepare the recipient list in advance and have the message set up so all you need to enter are the birth details and a couple of photos. Discuss with your partner who should be on the list. It helps to prepare this in advance, as it's one less thing to think about following the birth of your baby, and there's less of a chance you'll forget to add certain people.

• • ♦ • •

366 Sterilize pump parts, bottles, and pacifiers. There will be a lot to do when you return home with your baby. You will not want to be standing in the kitchen with a crying baby, figuring out how to sterilize important baby gear. This can all be done before the baby is born. Always read product directions to ensure you are properly sterilizing the items. One common way to sterilize products is with boiling water. Place (disassembled) items in a pot with water. Bring water to a boil, keep products in the boiling water for five minutes, and then remove with clean tongs. Make sure to keep items in a clean and clear area so they will be ready for use.

367 Go on day care tours and put your name on waitlists. Depending on where you live, childcare can be a competitive situation. Some parents will get their kids on a waitlist before they are born. If this is the case in your area, go on tours and put your name on waitlists early to avoid scrambling for care later.

• • ♦ • •

368 Book a newborn photoshoot and plan your outfits. If you want to commemorate your newborn's first weeks, schedule this photoshoot in advance. Research and speak with photographers to find one that you like, and have a loose appointment set. To capture the sleepiest newborn pictures, aim to have them taken within the first two weeks following birth. In addition to booking the photographer, plan outfits for your whole family. Remember that within two weeks of delivery your body will not be back to its pre-pregnancy size. Look through your favorite maternity items and select one or two to have washed and ready for the shoot.

369 Call your insurance to get a breast pump, or purchase one on your own, before the baby arrives. If you're planning to pump, it's great to get a pump before the baby arrives. Many insurance plans cover this, so take the time to call your insurance company and find out what is covered and what your options are. By getting it in advance, you'll have time to read about how to use it before it's go time.

••✦••

370 Create a diaper station (or multiple stations) in your house. If you live in a one-story home, one main diaper-changing station should be sufficient. If you live in a two- or more-story house, you may want to consider a mini station on each floor. This way, wherever you are with the baby, you can easily access the necessary supplies without going up and down the stairs.

••✦••

371 Place "baby essential" baskets around the house. Strategically set up baby essential baskets in favorite spots throughout your house so when you and the baby are cuddling up in your comfiest chair, whatever you need is within arm's reach. Include burp cloths, snacks (for you), and pacifiers in the basket.

372 Use a shower caddy to make a mobile nursing or bottle-feeding kit. Newborn babies eat frequently, and you may find yourself feeding them all over your house (in the living room, the nursery, your bedroom, etc.). If you'd prefer not to have stations set up all over your house, put the essentials that you will be using (such as a water bottle for you, burp cloth, etc.) in a shower caddy. This way you can easily carry your items around the house, ready to feed your baby wherever you are.

•••◆•••

373 Make a hair and nail appointment around thirty-five weeks. If it matters to you, go ahead and get pampered and prepped in your last month with hair and nail appointments. If this isn't important to you, skip it. It's also great to get these appointments out of the way in the final month of pregnancy because it will become tougher to find time for them in the first few weeks or months following your baby's arrival.

374 Write out a list of whom you want to come to the hospital. Make a plan with your partner of who will be present at the birth. Will you want members of your family in the delivery room, in the waiting room, or waiting at home? Decide what you are most comfortable with, and don't be worried about offending people. This is a big day for you, and you should be comfortable with the setup. Make sure your family members are aware of your plan so there aren't any surprises.

••◆••

375 Message friends and family about newborn visit protocol. Once you're home from the hospital, it's likely that friends and family will want to come by to meet the baby. Keep in mind that you will be recovering from childbirth. Figure out if and when you want people to visit, and set guidelines that work best for you. Send an email or text to these people so they know what to expect.

376 Decide when you will tell people you are in labor. Are you going to tell people as soon as you feel a contraction, or will you wait until you're admitted to the hospital? Or would you prefer to hold off on spreading the news until the baby has made their appearance? Make sure your partner or support person knows the plan so they can handle the communications.

• • ♦ • •

377 Request your maternity leave details in writing from work. Hopefully you have spoken with your boss and human resources and have hashed out the details of your maternity leave. As trusting as you are of the situation, don't only rely on what was said—get the details in writing as well. This will be helpful to refer to when your brain is feeling foggy during new mom life, or if your company is not adhering to the agreed-upon arrangement.

378 Make homemade padsicles to ease postpartum pains. These frozen pads will feel heavenly postbirth. Here's how to make them: Open up an overnight pad and lay it flat on a table (do not remove the adhesive backing). Spread a generous layer of aloe vera on the length of the pad. Next, pour witch hazel on top of the aloe vera. Finish it off with an optional drop of lavender essential oil. Make sure all ingredients are alcohol-free. Rewrap the pad, put it in a plastic bag, and place it in the freezer. Make eight for the first few postpartum days. When you return home from the hospital, you can put these into your underwear for cooling and soothing relief.

• • ♦ • •

379 Buy nursing pads or cotton rounds to stop milk stains. As your milk supply is established, it is common for your nipples to leak. This can happen during the end of pregnancy and while breastfeeding. You can choose disposable pads or washable pads, or you can even use cotton makeup rounds to stop the leaking before it gets to your shirt.

380 Mark in your calendar how you will split maternity and paternity leave. If you and your partner both have some sort of leave, decide how you're going to use the days. Will you be home together after the baby arrives? Or will you take turns; first you use your maternity leave, and then once you go back to work, your partner takes their leave? Figure out what works best for your situation, and mark it in a shared calendar.

◆

381 Buy overnight pads or adult diapers to have on hand for the first month postpartum. It's a no-brainer that your baby will need diapers—but there's also a good chance that you will need them as well. Heavy bleeding is normal after pregnancy and can last up to six weeks. You cannot use tampons during this time due to a risk of infection, so make sure you have a supply of high-absorbency pads, or instead buy adult diapers to wear.

382 Hold an ice cube to learn your labor coping mechanisms. There are a variety of ways to deal with labor pains. It's hard to know how you will respond until the time comes and you feel a real contraction, but here is a trick that can help you prepare. Contractions during the various stages of labor usually last somewhere between thirty and ninety seconds per contraction. To get an understanding of the most effective coping mechanisms for you, hold an ice cube in a closed fist for one minute (note: Do not try this exercise if you have Raynaud's disease, a condition in which blood vessels severely constrict when exposed to cold). Try a few different things to get through the cold discomfort. What makes you feel better or makes the time seem longer or shorter? Try counting, deep breaths, closing your eyes, visualizations, and focusing on one image. Does having your partner talk you through the minute make it go by faster or slower? Perhaps a shoulder massage helps. If something does seem to help, plan to use this technique during labor.

383 **Practice labor positions at home.** There are a wide variety of labor positions you can use to deal with the pain of labor and encourage the baby to descend. Don't wait until you're actually in labor to give these a try. Research and practice a handful of labor positions, figure out which ones you feel most comfortable with, and then you'll be ready to put these into use when you do go into labor. Try them with your partner so they know how to best assist you in these positions, and when things get tense as you're laboring, they can remind you of which positions might help.

• • ♦ • •

384 **Pretend you are blowing up a balloon to practice labor breathing.** Breathing seems like a simple enough task, but it's something you should practice for labor. One style of breathing that may help is to pretend you are blowing up a balloon. Begin with a relaxed face, breathe in through your nose, and exhale out through your mouth, as if you are blowing up a balloon. Do this while visualizing the balloon, and the visualization may take some focus off your pain while you are in labor.

385 Practice perineal massage to stretch your vagina in preparation for birth. As you head into the final weeks of pregnancy, you can perform gentle perineal massages that may help lessen the amount of tearing you experience during birth. Ask your doctor for specific advice on how to do this, and consider adding it to your routine when you are around thirty-four weeks pregnant.

••◆••

386 Look up *YouTube* workouts that induce labor. If you've reached your due date and you're getting antsy, there are some workouts and exercise moves that may help safely induce labor. Look up workouts online that are posted by certified professionals.

••◆••

387 Enjoy the ride! Finally, don't forget to enjoy this experience! Stay strong through the finish and remember to take in these incredible moments and celebrate what an amazing job you're doing.

PARTNER HACKS

Get Through the Home Stretch

388 **Schedule a haircut close to the due date.** Your baby won't be judging how shaggy your hair is, but it's nice to have a haircut close to your partner's due date so you can look put together in the first photos with the baby. And if you're planning to do a newborn photoshoot, you'll be ready and won't have to rush to the barber in those first two weeks with the baby.

389 **Program important numbers into your phone and know whom to call.** Important numbers include the hospital or nurse hotline for when your partner goes into labor, and important family numbers, like your partner's parents if she wants them to be kept up to date on the labor status.

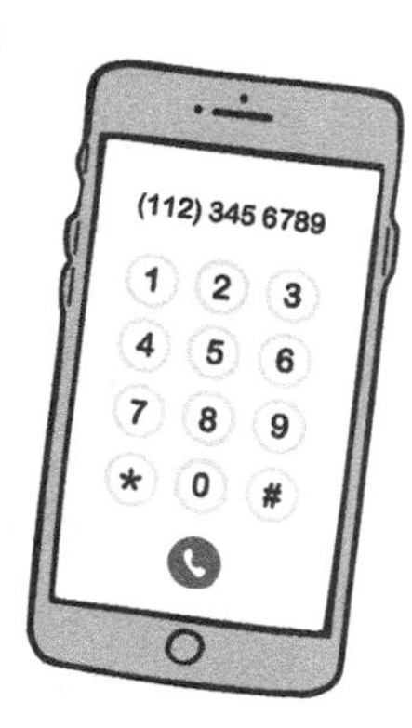

390 **Pack your own hospital bag with your essentials.** Your partner is busy packing her own, and probably the baby's, bag for the hospital, so make sure you pack your own bag and that it's ready to go in those final weeks leading up to the due date. Consider packing a pillow and blanket, a change of clothes, snacks and drinks (caffeinated drinks are a good choice; it can be a long experience), charging cords, a camera, and any other essentials that you might need for a two- or three-day stay at the hospital, especially if the hospital isn't very close to your home.

391 **Pay close attention during the hospital tour and take notes in your phone.** Your partner probably has a ton on her mind, and even if she pays attention during the hospital tour, you are responsible for paying even closer attention. When your partner does go into labor, she won't be thinking about where to park or check in; she's going to be focused on breathing through her contractions. It's up to you to know all these details, so make sure you're paying attention during the tour and will know what to do when the time comes. Take notes in your phone or on a notepad so you don't forget.

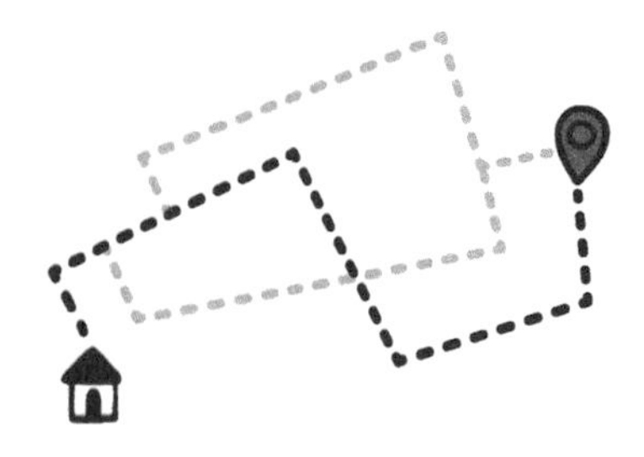

392 **Make note of the traffic and possible routes to the hospital.** Unless your partner is having a scheduled C-section, it's impossible to know when she will go into labor, and also impossible to know what the traffic will be like getting to the hospital. Be as prepared as possible by checking traffic during different times of day leading up to the due date. Think about how rush hour could change your best route. Have a game plan ready to put into action.

393 **Download a contraction tracking app.** Once your partner begins having contractions, you'll want to start timing them, both how long each contraction lasts and how long it is between contractions. There are free apps you can have on your phone to help with the timing. Download one of these ahead of time so you're ready to jump into action once the contractions begin.

394 **Purchase or make your own massage supplies with common household items.** Childbirth isn't a relaxing experience, but providing a gentle massage for your partner may make it a little bit better. Be prepared with a few special items to improve your massage skills. You can purchase handheld massage tools (battery operated or not) or create your own massage tools. Two simple examples are placing two tennis balls in a tube sock or filling a water bottle with warm water that you can use to roll up and down your partner's back.

395 **Fill your gas tank whenever you are as low as a quarter full.** As the due date nears, make sure your car is never approaching an empty gas tank. Your laboring partner will likely not appreciate a stop at the gas station on the way to the hospital.

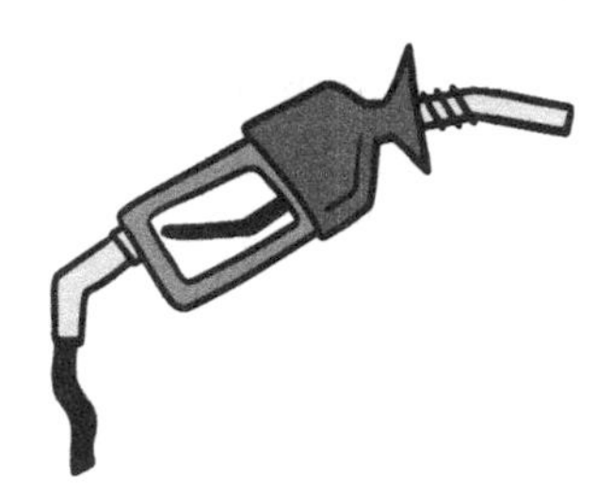

396 **Look up delivery food options near the hospital to prepare for the first meal after the baby arrives.** There have been a lot of off-limit foods for your partner during pregnancy, so once the baby arrives, it's time to give in to those cravings. Plus, labor is exhausting, and your partner will likely be very hungry after it's over. Check delivery food options near the hospital, and figure out what your partner will want so you can take care of the ordering for the big post-labor meal.

397 **Discuss and write down the photo plan for labor and look on *Pinterest* for creative ways to capture the event.** Does your partner want photos taken while in labor? Or maybe only following the labor? Know what she wants so you can be ready to appropriately capture it. Have her think about if there are certain photos or elements that she would like documented, and keep a list of these in the Notes app of your phone. Do your own brainstorming as well and be ready to capture the special and unique elements of your child's birth.

398 **Review your partner's birth preferences plan and know how to advocate for her.** Childbirth is an emotional ride, and your partner will have a lot on her plate when she's in labor. It may be hard for her to voice her opinions or to ask for the things that she needs. And as her support person, that's where you come in. She should be able to lean on you, both leading up to the labor, while in labor, and following the birth. Make sure you have enough discussions ahead of time to know how you can help her in the process and what choices are most important to her. The more you talk about it and the more open you are with each other, the better you will be able to support her when she needs it most. Know what's on your partner's birth preferences plan and be able to talk through elements at the hospital.

399 **Stay calm.** Now that you've made it through these nine months supporting your partner, continue to stay calm and to support her as much as possible in the final days leading up to, during, and after labor.

INDEX